Adam Held

HCG Diet Simplified

Strategies, Phases, and Results

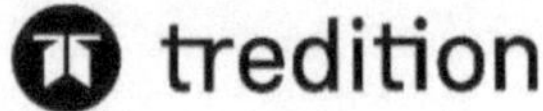

Druck und Distribution im Auftrag des Autors:
tredition GmbH, Heinz-Beusen-Stieg 5, 22926 Ahrensburg, Deutschland

Disclaimer

It is important to note that the information contained in this book is just intended for informational reasons and does not constitute professional, nutritional, or medical advice. The writers and publishers of this book do not accept any responsibility for any loss, damage, or harm that may be incurred as a consequence of the implementation of the strategies, procedures, or recommendations that are detailed in this book.

Prior to commencing any diet or nutrition program, it is strongly recommended that you get the advice of a trained physician or nutritionist. This will allow you to assess whether or not the strategies given in this book are suitable for your specific requirements. Various diets and supplements have different effects on different people because every body is different.

The reader is responsible for carrying out the advice and recommendations included in this book in a responsible manner and making a decision based on accurate information while doing so. It is strongly advised that the instructions and guidelines provided by competent professionals be adhered to, and that the right specialists be consulted in the event that any problems or queries occur.

Each and every attempt has been made by the authors and publishers of this book to guarantee that the material that is included in this book is correct and up to date. On the other hand, they are unable to ensure that the information that is provided is accurate, full, or at the appropriate time.

Every reader is accountable for his or her own choices and actions, and they are expected to take full responsibility for how the information offered in this book is applied in their own lives. In the event that any damage or loss occurs, whether it be direct or indirect, as a consequence of the execution of the methods or procedures discussed in this book, neither the authors nor the publishers of this book can be held liable for any compensation.

Additionally, it is recommended that the material contained in this book be verified with other reliable sources, and that specific requirements and circumstances be taken into consideration. Using the material that is provided in this book is done so at your own discretion and risk.

Take into consideration that the HCG diet is not appropriate for everyone, and that individual requirements, health issues, and medical conditions may all play a role in the decision-making process. A certified nutritionist or physician should be consulted prior to beginning any kind of diet or nutrition program. This is a strongly advised course of action.

Contents

Introduction

Throughout the course of this book, I will provide you with all of the information you require to comprehend and successfully implement the HCG diet, as well as help you on your journey to effective weight loss.

At the outset, I would like to present you with the HCG diet as the first topic of discussion. What exactly is the HCG diet, and what are the goals of the diet, will be explained to you. It is essential that you have a complete comprehension of what to anticipate and the advantages that this diet may provide when you begin it.

We will now delve even further into the scientific rationale behind the HCG diet. In this lesson, you will learn about the function of the hormone human chorionic gonadotropin (HCG) in the body as well as the part it plays in the process of weight reduction. In this section, we will examine the scientific evidence and research that substantiates the efficacy of the HCG diet.

For you to be able to successfully adopt the HCG diet, it is essential that you have a solid understanding of how it operates. In this section, we will examine the various phases of the diet in great detail and provide a step-by-step explanation of what to look for during each phase. To assist you in accomplishing your weight loss objectives, you will be provided with specific instructions and useful advice.

In addition, this book provides answers to frequently asked questions, which will let you address any issues you might have and provide you with a thorough grasp of the HCG diet regime. You will have an understanding of the most effective ways to be ready for the diet, as well as the way in which it might improve your health.

The fact that you have decided to go with the HCG diet and are prepared to make some great changes in your life is very exciting to me. With the assistance of this detailed guide, you will be able to properly execute the HCG diet and accomplish your objectives regarding weight loss. Are you prepared to embark on this thrilling adventure? In that case, let's embark on a journey together into the realm of the HCG diet!

Chapter 1: Basics of the HCG diet

1.1 History of the HCG diet

The HCG diet has a long and lengthy history that dates back many years. Over the course of the 1950s, Dr. Albert T. W. Simeons was the one who initially invented it. Dr. Simeons made the discovery that the hormone human chorionic gonadotropin (HCG), which is released during pregnancy, can have beneficial effects on the metabolism and the burning of fat.

In his pursuit of knowledge on the efficacy of the HCG diet, Dr. Simeons carried out a great number of tests and experiments. A low-calorie diet plus the administration of HCG injections led to significant weight loss, particularly in troublesome areas such as the hips, thighs, and belly, according to his findings. He discovered that this combination resulted in significant weight loss.

Over the course of the subsequent decades, the HCG diet became increasingly well-known and was utilized by a large number of individuals as an efficient strategy for shedding excess pounds. In spite of the fact that the HCG diet has been the subject of debates and debates in the past, it continues to be a popular choice among those who are interested in reducing their weight.

In this chapter, you will not only learn about the historical context of the HCG diet, but you will also learn about significant milestones and developments that have occurred over the course of the years. As time goes on, you will observe how the HCG diet has developed into a more holistic approach to weight management and how it has grown over time.

The history of the HCG diet is fascinating, and it demonstrates that it is not just a passing trend; rather, it is founded on solid scientific principles and a significant amount of research that has been conducted over a period of many years. It has assisted a great number of individuals in accomplishing their weight loss objectives and leading healthier lives.

Are you prepared to go deeper into the history of the HCG diet and establish the groundwork for your own successful weight loss journey? If that is the case, then let us proceed together and find out more fascinating information in the following area!

1.2 What is HCG?

Inside this part, I will provide a comprehensive explanation of what HCG is and the function it serves within the HCG diet.

The abbreviation HCG refers to human chorionic gonadotropin, which is a hormone that is created by the body on its own initiative, particularly during pregnancy. The placenta is responsible for its production, and its primary function is to get the body ready to meet the requirements of the developing embryo.

Within the context of the HCG diet, this hormone is administered in the form of injections, drops, or tablets. The theory behind it is that HCG has an effect on the metabolism and increases the amount of fat that is burned. Supplementation with HCG encourages the body to draw upon its fat reserves in order to satisfy its energy requirements. Consequently, this makes it possible to lose weight effectively, particularly in troublesome areas such as the hips, thighs, and belly.

Understand that HCG is not the only factor responsible for weight loss. This is a vital point to keep in mind. Instead, it serves as a supplement to the low-calorie diet that is taken during the phase of the HCG diet that is being followed. In order to acquire the best possible outcomes, it is essential to combine the particular diet with the use of HCG.

Injections, drops, and pills are some of the numerous ways that HCG can be administered during pregnancy. Each approach comes with its own set of benefits and drawbacks, and you are free to select the approach that caters to your requirements and preferences the most effectively. Before beginning the HCG diet, it is essential to conduct exhaustive study on the various options available to you and, if further information is required, to consult with a healthcare practitioner.

For the purpose of assisting you in selecting the HCG method that is most suitable for you, this chapter will provide you with comprehensive information regarding the various HCG products and forms. You will also gain an understanding of the fundamentals of how the hormone HCG operates within the body and the advantages it provides for weight loss.

Have you reached the point where you are prepared to go deeper into the world of HCG and comprehend how this hormone contributes to the HCG diet? Then, let's proceed together and check out the following part to find out more about the function of HCG in the process of weight reduction!

1.3 HCG products and forms

In this section, we will examine the various HCG products and forms in greater detail than it was previously discussed.

During the HCG diet, there are a few different ways that HCG can be administered. Injectables, drops, and tablets are the most prevalent means of administration. Considering that every one of these kinds comes with its own set of benefits and drawbacks, it is essential to select the one that caters to your requirements and preferences the most effectively.

- Injections: HCG can be administered in the form of injections. These are usually given subcutaneously, i.e. under the skin. The advantages of injections are rapid absorption of the hormone into the body and accurate dosing. However, it requires some practice and may require guidance or assistance from a healthcare professional.
- Drops: HCG drops are a popular alternative to injections. They are taken orally and can be used conveniently at home. The advantages of HCG drops are their simplicity and the ability to use them independently. However, it is important to obtain high-quality drops from trusted sources and follow the instructions carefully.
- Tablets: HCG tablets are another option for delivering the hormone. They are also taken orally and offer ease of use. However, it is important to note that HCG in tablet form may not be as effective as in the other forms. Again, it's crucial to choose high-quality tablets from trusted providers and follow the instructions carefully.

In the following chapter, you will be provided with in-depth information regarding the benefits and drawbacks associated with each HCG type. It will be explained to you in a variety of ways, and you will be able to determine which of these methods is most suitable for you. Before beginning the HCG diet, it is strongly recommended that you conduct exhaustive study on the various options available to you and, if required, seek the advice of a qualified medical practitioner.

Are you prepared to acquire knowledge about the various HCG products and forms, and to make a decision regarding your HCG diet that is based on accurate information? Next, let's go on together and take a more in-depth look at the role that HCG plays in the process of weight loss in the following part!

1.4 The role of HCG in weight loss

In the following paragraphs, we will examine the function of HCG in the process of weight loss in greater depth.

The hormone human chorionic gonadotropin, also known as HCG, is an essential component of the HCG diet and significantly impacts the process of weight loss in a number of different ways.

- Stimulation of metabolism: HCG can stimulate the metabolism, which leads to the body burning more energy, effectively reducing fat. HCG supplementation optimizes metabolism, resulting in increased fat burning, even on a low calorie diet.
- Preservation of muscle mass: During a low-calorie diet, there is often a risk that the body will not only lose fat, but also muscle mass. HCG helps to minimize muscle loss by stimulating the body to make increased use of fat reserves and to preserve muscle mass. This is especially important for achieving healthy and sustainable weight loss.
- Reducing hunger pangs: One of the challenges of a low-calorie diet is the constant feeling of hunger and cravings. HCG can help reduce hunger pangs and better control food cravings. This allows dieters to more easily stick to the prescribed diet and maintain the calorie deficit.

- Targeted fat burning: HCG diet aims to target stubborn fat deposits in the body, especially in problematic areas such as hips, thighs and abdomen. HCG helps put the body into fat burning mode and effectively tap into fat reserves.

HCG is not the only factor that contributes to weight loss; this is an essential point to keep in mind. To attain the best possible outcomes, it is necessary to combine the use of HCG with a diet that is low in calories. Not only does HCG assist the body in achieving the ideal weight, but it also assists in the maintenance of muscle mass and boosts the metabolism.

In this chapter, you will acquire additional knowledge regarding the unique role that HCG plays in the process of weight loss. The effects of HCG on the body, as well as the advantages it provides, will be explained to you. It is essential to have this knowledge in order to successfully adhere to the HCG diet and attain the best possible outcomes.

Have you reached the point where you are prepared to delve deeper into the HCG diet and investigate the role that HCG plays in weight loss in greater detail? In that case, let's proceed together and proceed to the following part to learn about the various phases of the HCG diet!

1.5 The different phases of the HCG diet

A comprehensive review of the HCG diet will be provided to you in this section, during which we will discuss the various phases of the diet.

There are multiple phases that make up the HCG diet, and each of these phases has its own set of objectives and prerequisites. To attain the best possible outcomes, it is essential to have a solid understanding of these stages and to proceed through them in the appropriate sequence.

- Loading phase: The loading phase, often referred to as the "loading phase", is about supplying the body with sufficient nutrients and replenishing fat reserves before the actual diet begins. During this phase, you eat high-calorie and high-fat foods to stimulate the metabolism and prepare the body for weight loss.

- Weight loss phase: The weight loss phase is the core of the HCG diet. During this phase, one follows a very low calorie diet, usually limited to 500-800 calories per day. At the same time, HCG is supplied to boost metabolism and make the body access fat reserves more. This phase usually lasts about 3-6 weeks, but can vary depending on the individual goal and plan.

- Stabilization phase: The weight loss phase is followed by the stabilization phase, which serves to maintain the weight achieved and prepare the body for a permanent change in diet. In this phase, calorie intake is slowly increased, but still within a controlled range. It is important to continue making healthy choices and maintaining a balanced diet during this phase.

- Maintenance phase: The maintenance phase is the last phase of the HCG diet. Here, the goal is to maintain the new eating habits and maintain the weight loss in the long term. In this phase, calorie intake is further adjusted and regular exercise and healthy food choices are recommended.

As you progress through this chapter, you will receive an in-depth summary of each stage of the HCG diet. It will be clear to you what the objective of each phase is, as well as the steps that you need to follow in order to effectively progress through the phases. To ensure that you are able to make the most of your HCG diet and face the hurdles that come with each phase, we will also provide you with particular guidance and tips.

Are you prepared to acquire knowledge on the many stages of the HCG diet and to build a comprehensive strategy for your weight loss objectives? Then, let's proceed together and find out some essential information regarding the phases of the HCG diet in the following part!

Chapter 2: Preparation for the HCG diet

2.1 Preparation for the diet

In this chapter, we will discuss the crucial part of getting ready for the HCG diet, which is the preparation phase.

In order to ensure that your weight loss efforts are successful, it is essential that you get yourself ready for the HCG diet. You will be able to adjust both psychologically and physically to the impending diet with the assistance of excellent preparation, which will allow you to obtain the greatest results possible.

- Educate yourself: Educate yourself thoroughly about the HCG diet, its principles and guidelines. Learn how it works, what foods are allowed and what restrictions there are. It is important to have a clear understanding of the diet in order to implement it successfully.
- Consult a professional: It may be helpful to consult with a medical professional, such as a doctor or nutritionist, before starting the

HCG diet. They can consider your individual needs and health goals and give you valuable advice.

- Prepare your body: Consider detoxifying your body in a healthy way before starting the HCG diet. For example, you could reduce your consumption of sugary drinks and processed foods and instead switch to a balanced diet with plenty of fruits, vegetables and whole grains.
- Create a supportive environment: Share your plan to go on the HCG diet with your social circle. Explain to them why weight loss is important to you and how they can support you. This can help gain support and understanding and make it easier for you to stay motivated during the diet.
- Prepare your meals: Plan ahead and prepare your meals, especially for the weight loss period. Think about healthy recipes, make a shopping plan and prepare some meals in advance if necessary. This will make it easier for you to stick to the food you are given during the diet.
- Create a positive mindset: Approach the HCG diet with a positive mindset. Visualize your desired outcome and remind yourself

regularly why you are undertaking this journey. Set realistic goals and encourage yourself to persevere during the diet.

It is essential to get ready for the HCG diet in order to have a great beginning. Through the process of educating yourself, preparing your body, cultivating a supportive environment, and having a positive mindset, you will lay the groundwork for your success in losing weight.

Would you be willing to put in a lot of effort to get ready for the HCG diet and attain the greatest possible results? After that, let's go on to the following part and discuss some other significant areas of preparation together!

2.2 Shopping list and stockpiling

As part of the HCG diet, we will discuss the process of creating a shopping list and stocking up on the necessary items.

For the purpose of ensuring that you always have the appropriate meals on hand and achieving success while following the HCG diet, it is essential to have a well-planned grocery list and to stock up carefully.

- Create a shopping list: Start by making a comprehensive shopping list for the HCG diet. Take into account the foods that are allowed and the recipes that you want to use. Make sure you have all the necessary ingredients for your meals and snacks on the list.
- Choose fresh foods: Focus on fresh, unprocessed foods. Fill your cart with a variety of vegetables and fruits, lean meats, fish, eggs and low-fat dairy products. Avoid processed foods, sugary products and foods high in fat.
- Pay attention to portion sizes: When compiling your shopping list, keep in mind the recommended portion sizes for the HCG diet. It is important to keep track of calorie intake and consume the right amount of food to achieve the desired results.
- Keep your supplies stocked: Regularly check and replenish your supplies to ensure you always have the right foods on hand. Keep your kitchen well stocked to avoid

temptations and easily access the foods you are allowed.

- Organize your fridge: Rearrange your fridge so that HCG-friendly foods are easily accessible. Separate them from unhealthy foods to avoid distractions. Make it a habit to organize your supplies and make sure you always have the right foods on hand.

It will be much simpler for you to adhere to the guidelines that have been established throughout the HCG diet if you have a well-planned grocery list and carefully stockpile your supplies. You can establish an environment that is conducive to your healthy weight reduction by stocking up on food, selecting foods that are both fresh and nutritious, and maintaining an organized refrigerator.

In preparation for the HCG diet, are you prepared to create a comprehensive shopping list and stock up on the necessary supplies? If that is the case, then let us proceed together and investigate further significant areas of preparation in the following part!

2.3 Mental preparation

The mental preparation for the HCG diet is going to be the topic of discussion in this section. This is due to the fact that the success of a diet is dependent not only on the physical, but also on the mental attitude as well.

- Set clear goals: Define clear and realistic goals for your weight loss. Visualize how you want to feel and look at the end of the diet. Write down your goals and read them regularly to keep yourself motivated.
- Positive Affirmations: Use positive affirmations to strengthen your mental attitude. Repeat positive phrases such as "I am in control of my diet" or "I can achieve my goals." By cultivating positive thoughts, you can strengthen your motivation and willpower.
- Coping strategies: Develop strategies to deal with challenges while dieting. Identify potential obstacles and find solutions to deal with them. This may include distracting yourself with unhealthy foods at the office or coping with emotional eating bouts.
- Visualize success: Use the power of visualization to support your success during the

diet. Vividly imagine yourself reaching your goal weight, feeling energized and confident. Visualize yourself making healthy choices and celebrating your progress.

- Reward yourself: Set milestones and reward yourself for your progress. Plan small rewards for each success you achieve, whether it's a relaxing massage, a new book, or some other form of self-care. These rewards can help keep you motivated and give you positive reinforcement.
- Seek support: find a support group or partners with whom you can interact and share experiences. This can be in the form of friends, family members or online communities. The support of others can help you get through difficult times and encourage you to stick to your goals.

In order to be successful with the HCG diet, mental preparation is just as vital as physical preparation. You can lay the groundwork for a good and effective weight loss by establishing crystal-clear goals, employing positive mantras, developing coping skills, visualizing accomplishment, rewarding yourself, and seeking help.

Do you feel that you are ready to psychologically prepare yourself for the HCG diet and cultivate a strong mental attitude? After that, let's go on to the following part and discuss some other significant areas of preparation together!

2.4 Objective and motivation

In this section we will look at goal setting and motivation, as they play a crucial role in the successful implementation of the HCG diet.

- Set clear and realistic goals: Define your goals for the HCG diet clearly and precisely. Do you want to lose a certain number of kilograms or feel better in your body? Be realistic in setting goals and take into account factors such as your starting weight, your health and your lifestyle.
- Express your goals: Write down your goals and make them visible. Write them down on a piece of paper and hang it somewhere

you'll see it every day, such as the refrigerator or bathroom mirror. Visually reminding yourself of your goals can help you stay focused and motivate you.

- Find your motivation: Think about why you want to do the HCG diet and what motivates you. Do you want to feel better in your body, improve your health or have more energy? Identify your personal motivators and keep them present during the diet.

- Keep a diary: Keep a diary in which you record your progress, thoughts and feelings during the HCG diet. Write down how you feel after meals, what challenges you overcome and what successes you achieve. The diary can help you stay on track and keep you motivated.

- Visualize your success: Vividly imagine how you will feel when you have achieved your goals. Visualize yourself with more confidence, in a healthier body, and with a positive attitude toward food and exercise. This visual imagination can boost your motivation and remind you why you are doing the HCG diet.

- Reward yourself for milestones: Set intermediate goals and reward yourself when you reach them. Plan small rewards like a spa weekend, new clothes or a pampering treatment. These rewards validate your efforts and keep your motivation high.

Maintaining your motivation throughout the HCG diet and increasing your chances of success can be accomplished by establishing goals that are both specific and attainable, determining what motivates you, keeping a journal, visualizing yourself succeeding, and rewarding yourself for reaching different milestones along the way.

Are you prepared to establish your objectives and discover the motivation you need to achieve success on the HCG diet? After that, let's go on to the following part and discuss some other significant areas of preparation together!

2.5 Physical activity during the HCG diet

We are going to devote this section to discussing the significance of engaging in physical activity while following the HCG regime.

When it comes to making progress toward your weight reduction goals and enhancing your overall health, physical activity is an essential component. Even while the HCG diet restricts the number of calories you consume, this does not mean that you should go absolutely easy on yourself. Integrating exercise into your routine will help you achieve better outcomes and tone your body.

When engaging in physical activity while adhering to the HCG diet, it is essential to keep the following critical considerations in mind:

- Consult a professional: Before you begin any new exercise program, you should consult with a medical professional, such as a doctor or trainer. They can give you recommendations on what types of exercises are best suited to your fitness level and goals.

- Choose appropriate activities: Choose activities that you enjoy and that fit your fitness level. This could be walking, cycling, swimming or yoga. Find activities that motivate you and that you can do regularly.
- Pay attention to your limits: Listen to your body and watch your limits. During the HCG diet, you may have less energy than usual. Adjust your training accordingly and make sure you don't overexert yourself.
- Consider interval training: Interval training, where you combine short, intense exercises with short recovery periods, can be an effective way to burn calories and improve your fitness. Talk to a trainer about incorporating interval training into your exercise program.
- Stay active in everyday life: In addition to planned workouts, it is important to stay active in everyday life. Take every opportunity to move, such as climbing stairs instead of taking elevators, taking short walks during your lunch break, or gardening.
- Listen to your body: During the HCG diet it is especially important to pay attention to your body's needs. If you feel tired or exhausted, take time to rest and recover. Listen

to your body's signals and adjust your training accordingly.

In addition to assisting you in losing weight while on the HCG diet, engaging in physical activity can also improve your overall health and well-being. Spend time engaging in activities that are both enjoyable and inspiring, maintain an active lifestyle, and make it a point to pay attention to the requirements of your body.

Are you prepared to participate in physical activity as part of your HCG diet and to enjoy the advantages that come with physical activity? After that, let's go on to the following part and discuss some other significant areas of preparation together!

Chapter 3: Phase 1 - The loading or preparation phase

3.1 The importance of the loading phase

In the following chapter, we will discuss the loading or preparation phase of the HCG diet, which is the initial step of the diet regime.

The loading phase is an essential step in the process of getting the body ready for the weight loss that is to come. Your primary focus during this period is on ensuring that your body receives an adequate amount of nutrients and that your energy reserves are replenished. The following are some crucial considerations to keep in mind throughout the loading phase:

- Increase your calorie intake: During the loading phase, you should increase your calorie intake to replenish your energy reserves. Focus on high-calorie, healthy foods such as avocados, nuts, seeds, fatty fish and whole grains. However, avoid fatty and sugary foods.

- Eat enough healthy fats: Healthy fats are important during the loading phase to provide your body with energy. Add foods like olive oil, coconut oil, avocados and nuts to your diet. Make sure you still maintain a balanced diet and don't consume overly fatty foods.

- Avoid alcohol and sugary drinks: During the loading phase you should avoid alcohol and sugary drinks. These can interfere with your efforts to prepare for the HCG diet. Instead, drink plenty of water, herbal teas and unsweetened beverages to keep your body hydrated.

- Plan your meals: It is important to plan your meals well during the loading phase. Prepare meals that are rich in protein, healthy carbohydrates and healthy fats. Structure your meals so that you get enough energy and feel full.

- Reduce stress: Stress can have a negative impact on the preparation phase. Try to minimize stress factors and integrate relaxation techniques such as meditation, yoga or walks into your daily routine. A stress-free preparation phase can help you focus on the upcoming phases of the HCG diet.

As a crucial component of the HCG diet, the loading phase is designed to provide your body with the optimal preparation for the subsequent weight reduction. You may create the groundwork for the success of the HCG diet by increasing the number of calories you consume, incorporating healthy fats in your diet, avoiding consume alcohol and sugary drinks, organizing your meals, and lowering the amount of stress you experience.

Do you feel that you are prepared to transition into the loading phase of the HCG diet and get your body ready in the most effective way possible? Then, in the following section, let's go over some additional information about the loading process alongside one another!

3.2 Guidelines and strategies for the loading phase

The purpose of this part is to provide you with the most comprehensive preparation possible for beginning the HCG diet by discussing the guidelines and tactics for the loading phase.

When you are in the loading phase of the HCG diet, you are supplying your body with sufficient amounts of nutrients and energy reserves so that it may effectively finish the subsequent phases of the diet. The loading phase is characterized by the following fundamental rules and techniques that must be adhered to:

- Increase your calorie intake: During the loading phase, it is important to increase your calorie intake to provide your body with enough energy. Focus on high calorie foods such as nuts, seeds, fatty fish, whole grains and healthy oils. However, make sure you still maintain a balanced diet and don't consume excessively fatty or sugary foods.
- Choose healthy foods: During the loading phase, choose healthy and nutrient-rich foods to provide your body with the nutrients it needs. Add fruits, vegetables, lean meats, fish, eggs, dairy products and whole grains to your diet. These foods provide essential nutrients and keep you full.
- Avoid fatty and sugary foods: Although you are increasing your calorie intake, it is

important to avoid fatty and sugary foods during the loading phase. These foods can lead to weight gain and an unhealthy metabolism. Instead, focus on healthy, natural foods that provide your body with essential nutrients.

- Drink enough water: During the loading phase, it is important to drink enough water to keep your body hydrated and flush out toxins. Drink at least 8 glasses of water per day and avoid sugary drinks. Water also helps control your hunger pangs and keep you full.
- Plan your meals: Plan your meals in advance during the loading phase to ensure you get a balanced diet. Consider all major nutrient groups such as proteins, carbohydrates, fats, vitamins and minerals. Structure your meals so that they fill you up and keep your energy levels stable.
- Avoid alcohol and sugary drinks: During the loading phase you should avoid alcohol and sugary drinks. Alcohol contains empty calories and can interfere with your efforts to prepare for the HCG diet. Drink water, herbal teas or unsweetened beverages instead.

When it comes to getting your body ready for the HCG diet, the loading phase is a very essential time. You may lay the groundwork for a good beginning to the HCG diet by increasing the number of calories you consume, selecting nutritious foods, avoiding foods that are high in fat and sugar, drinking an adequate amount of water, organizing your meals, and putting an end to alcohol consumption.

Are you prepared to put into action the recommendations and methods that are associated with the loading phase and to get yourself ready for the beginning of the HCG diet in the best possible way? Then, in the following section, let's go over some additional information concerning the Loading Phase alongside one another!

3.3 Foods recommended during the loading phase

During the loading phase, eating the foods that are recommended will be the topic of discussion in this section. In order to ensure that your body is in the best possible condition for the subsequent phases of the HCG diet, these foods will supply it with the essential nutrients it needs. The following is a list of meals that are suggested to be consumed during the loading phase:

- Nuts and seeds: Nuts and seeds are an excellent source of healthy fats, vitamins and minerals. Almonds, walnuts, chia seeds and flax seeds are just a few examples of nutrient-rich options. You can enjoy them as a snack or incorporate them into your meals.
- Avocados: Avocados are rich in healthy fats, fiber and nutrients. They can add a creamy texture to your salads, smoothies or sandwiches. Avocados also contain antioxidants that are good for your health.
- Fatty fish: Fatty fish like salmon, mackerel and tuna are rich in omega-3 fatty acids, which have anti-inflammatory properties and are good for your cardiovascular system. Add them to your meals to reap their health benefits.
- Whole grain products: Whole grain products such as oatmeal, quinoa and whole wheat bread are rich in fiber and provide long-lasting energy. They can serve as the basis for a balanced meal and keep you full longer.

- Lean meat and poultry: Lean meat and poultry are a good source of protein during the loading phase. Chicken breast, turkey breast, lean beef and lean pork are options that are low in fat but still provide high-quality protein.
- Eggs: Eggs are rich in protein and contain many important nutrients. They can be prepared in different ways, such as boiled, fried or as an omelet. Eggs are versatile and can be enjoyed at any meal.
- Dairy products: Low-fat dairy products such as yogurt, cheese and low-fat milk can be consumed during the loading phase. They contain protein and calcium, which is important for your bone health.

It is essential to take note that the foods that are recommended to be consumed during the loading phase are nutritious and abundant in nutrients. You should steer clear of foods that are high in fat and sugar because they do not adequately prepare your body for the HCG diet.

It is possible to ensure that your body receives the nutrients it requires and that you feel your best during the preparation phase of the HCG diet by include foods such as nuts, seeds, avocados, fatty fish, whole grains, lean meats, poultry, eggs, and dairy products in your diet.

Are you prepared to incorporate these items into your diet during the loading period so that you may get your body ready in the most effective way possible? Therefore, let's go on to the following section, where we will delve more into the loading phase of the HCG diet, and get ready for the subsequent phases of the diet regimen!

3.4 Foods that should be avoided

In this part of the article, we will discuss the foods that you should steer clear of while you are in the loading period. The consumption of these items may have a detrimental impact on your health and may also have an impact on the success of your preparation period. A number of foods, including those listed below, should be avoided during the loading phase:

- Fatty foods: Fatty foods such as fried foods, fast foods, fatty meats and foods high in

saturated fats should be avoided. These
foods contain high amounts of unhealthy fats
that can affect your health.

- Sugary foods and drinks: Sugary foods and
  drinks such as sodas, candy, cakes, cookies
  and ice cream should be avoided during the
  loading phase. These foods contain empty
  calories and can lead to weight gain.
- Alcohol: Alcoholic beverages should be
  avoided during the loading phase. Alcohol
  contains many calories and can hinder your
  efforts to prepare for the HCG diet. In addition, alcohol impairs your metabolic processes and can lead to dehydration.
- White flour products: White flour products
  such as white bread, pasta and baked goods
  should be reduced or avoided. These foods
  contain refined carbohydrates that can lead
  to a rapid rise in blood sugar levels.
- Processed foods: Processed foods such as fro-
  zen meals, snacks, ready meals and foods
  with many additives should be avoided.
  These foods often contain high amounts of
  salt, sugar, saturated fats and artificial ingredients.

- Sweeteners: Sweeteners such as aspartame, saccharin and sucralose should be avoided during the loading phase. They can cause cravings and increase your preference for sweet foods.

During the loading phase, it is essential to keep a balanced diet and to steer clear of things that can cause your body to experience stress or that can actually cause you to gain weight. You can build the groundwork for a successful preparation phase of the HCG diet by avoiding foods that are high in fat, foods and drinks that are high in sugar, alcohol, items made with white flour, processed foods, and sweets.

Do you feel prepared to steer clear of these meals throughout the loading phase and instead concentrate on maintaining a balanced diet? Therefore, let's go on to the following section, where we will delve more into the loading phase of the HCG diet, and get ready for the subsequent phases of the diet regimen!

3.5 Maintenance of metabolism during the loading phase

Within this part, we will discuss the various methods by which you can keep your metabolism going when you are in the loading period. If you want to successfully reduce weight and improve your health, having a metabolism that works properly is really necessary. The following are some essential pointers that will help you maintain a high metabolism during the loading phase:

- Regular meals: Eat regularly and plan your meals during the loading phase. It's important to provide your body with adequate energy while preventing cravings. Make sure you eat healthy, balanced meals, taking into account the recommended foods of the Loading Phase.
- Include proteins: Protein is essential for metabolism, as it increases the body's energy expenditure and helps build muscle. Therefore, incorporate protein-rich foods such as lean meats, poultry, fish, eggs, dairy products and plant-based protein sources into your meals.

- Staying active: Exercise and physical activity play an important role in maintaining metabolism. Engage in regular exercise such as walking, yoga, strength training or other activities you enjoy. This will help boost your metabolism and increase calories burned.
- Drink enough water: Adequate hydration is important for a well-functioning metabolism. Drink enough water to keep your body hydrated and metabolic processes running optimally. It is recommended to drink at least 8 glasses of water per day.
- Get enough sleep: Adequate sleep quality and duration are crucial for a healthy metabolism. Make sure to get enough sleep to rest and regenerate your body. Lack of sleep can slow metabolism and lead to weight gain.
- Stress management: Chronic stress can negatively affect metabolism. Find healthy ways to reduce stress, such as meditation, relaxation exercises, reading, or engaging in hobbies. By reducing stress, you promote a healthy metabolism.

By eating regular meals, including protein, staying active, drinking enough water, getting enough sleep and using stress management techniques, you can keep your metabolism optimal during the loading phase. This lays the foundation for a successful start to the HCG diet and effective weight loss.

Are you ready to implement these tips and support your metabolism during the loading phase? Therefore, let's go on to the following section, where we will delve more into the loading phase of the HCG diet, and get ready for the subsequent phases of the diet regimen!Maintaining a healthy metabolism during the loading period can be accomplished by consuming meals on a consistent basis, incorporating protein, remaining physically active, consuming a enough amount of water, obtaining sufficient sleep, and employing measures for stress management. This creates the groundwork for a good beginning to the HCG diet and for fat loss that is both efficient and effective.

Do you feel prepared to put these suggestions into action and provide your metabolism with help throughout the loading phase? Therefore, let's go on to the following section, where we will delve more into the loading phase of the HCG diet, and get ready for the subsequent phases of the diet regimen!

Chapter 4: Phase 2 - The Strictly Calorie Restricted Phase

4.1 The advantages of the calorie restricted phase

In this chapter, we will discuss phase 2 of the HCG diet, which is marked by a rigorous restriction on the number of calories that individual consumes. There are various advantages to your health and weight loss that come with the calorie restriction period, despite the fact that it can be difficult to go through. Following is a list of some of the most significant advantages:

- Effective weight loss: The calorie restricted phase allows for fast and effective weight loss. By reducing calorie intake, you force your body to access its fat reserves and use them as a source of energy. This allows you to make significant progress in your weight loss in a relatively short time.
- Reduction of hunger pangs: During the calorie-restricted phase, you may notice a reduced feeling of hunger. This is because HCG (human chorionic gonadotropin) helps regulate your appetite and increase your

feeling of fullness. This makes it easier for you to stick to the prescribed low-calorie diet.

- Preservation of muscle mass: Combining HCG with the calorie-restricted diet minimizes the loss of muscle mass. This is of great importance because muscle mass boosts metabolism and helps burn fat. By maintaining your muscle mass during the calorie-restricted phase, you support long-term weight loss and prevent the yo-yo effect.

- Improve insulin sensitivity: The calorie-restricted phase can help improve your insulin sensitivity. By reducing your intake of carbohydrates and focusing on a balanced diet, you can stabilize your blood sugar levels and optimize your body's insulin response. This has positive effects on metabolism and weight loss.

- Increase in energy level: Although the calorie-restricted phase involves a lower calorie intake, many people report an increased energy level during this phase. This may be due to the body accessing its fat reserves more and using them as a source of energy.

By providing your body with the right nutrients and maintaining a healthy, balanced
diet, you can keep your energy levels up.

While the phase of the HCG diet that involves restricting calories may be difficult to follow, it does
provide a lot of advantages for both your health and
your ability to lose weight. During this phase of the
HCG diet, there are numerous reasons to consider
doing so. Some of these reasons include effective
weight loss, a reduction in hunger pangs, the maintenance of muscle mass, and an improvement in insulin sensitivity.

Have you reached the point where you are prepared
to advance your weight reduction as well as savor
the benefits of the calorie-restricted phase? Find out
how you may effectively master phase 2 of the HCG
diet by reading the next part, which will provide you
with additional information regarding this phase of
the program.

4.2 Guidelines and strategies for phase 2

In the following section, we will discuss the essential principles and methods that are utilized during the second phase of the HCG diet. You will be able to successfully manage the phase of strictly limiting your calorie intake and obtain the best possible outcomes with the assistance of these suggestions and tactics. Listed below are some essential pointers:

- Follow the HCG diet protocols: Phase 2 of the HCG diet has specific protocols that you should follow. These include taking HCG daily, strictly following the calorie-restricted diet, and making the right food choices that are allowed. Strictly adhere to these protocols to achieve maximum results.
- Watch your calorie intake: During Phase 2 of the HCG diet, your daily calorie intake is usually between 500 and 800 calories. Make sure you stick to the recommended calorie levels to achieve effective weight loss. Plan your meals in advance to ensure you get enough nutrients while staying within the calorie restriction.

- Focus on protein-rich foods: Protein-rich foods play an important role in phase 2 of the HCG diet. They help maintain your muscles and promote a feeling of fullness. Incorporate lean meats, poultry, fish, eggs, and plant-based protein sources like tofu or legumes into your meals.

- Avoid fatty foods and sugary foods: During phase 2 of the HCG diet, you should avoid fatty foods and sugary foods. These foods contain a lot of calories and can hinder your weight loss. Instead, focus on healthy, low-fat options like lean meats, vegetables, fruits and low-fat dairy products.

- Pay attention to portion sizes: Even though calorie intake is limited in Phase 2, it's important to pay attention to portion sizes. Stick to the recommended amounts of foods allowed to ensure you get the right nutrients and meet your calorie goals.

- Drink enough water: Adequate hydration is important during phase 2 of the HCG diet. Drink enough water daily to keep your body hydrated and promote the elimination of toxins. This can also help reduce hunger pangs and support your metabolism.

- Stick to the recommended duration: Phase 2 of the HCG diet has a specific duration, which may vary depending on your individual goal and plan. Stick to the recommended duration to achieve optimal results and ensure the health of your body.

It is possible for you to successfully complete phase 2 of the HCG diet if you adhere to these instructions and implementation tactics. Be sure to adhere to the protocols, monitor your calorie intake, concentrate on foods that are high in protein, steer clear of foods that are high in fat and sugar, monitor the size of your portions, drink enough of water, and stay for the required amount of time. If you do things in this manner, you will establish the groundwork for successful weight loss and accomplish the outcomes you desire.

In order to move forward with Phase 2 of the HCG diet, are you prepared to put these rules and methods into action? Then, let's go on to the following section, where we will delve deeper into the specifics of Phase 2, and prepare ready for the subsequent phases!

4.3 HCG diet protocol

In the next section, we will examine the regimen for the HCG diet that is utilized throughout the second phase of the HCG diet journey. The regimen guarantees that you will acquire the finest outcomes possible and that you will enhance your weight loss efforts. According to the HCG diet program, the following are the most crucial aspects:

- Daily HCG intake: During phase 2 of the HCG diet it is important to take HCG daily. This can be in the form of HCG injections, HCG drops or HCG pellets. HCG intake supports weight loss, regulates appetite and helps maintain muscle mass.
- Calorie-restricted diet: The HCG diet protocol involves a strictly calorie-restricted diet. The daily calorie intake is usually between 500 and 800 calories. It is important to choose the foods allowed and carefully monitor calorie intake to achieve the desired result.
- Selection of allowed foods: During phase 2 of the HCG diet, there is a list of allowed foods that you can consume. These foods are low in calories, high in protein and low in fat. They

include lean meats, poultry, fish, seafood, vegetables, fruits and certain low-fat dairy products. Avoid foods that are not on the list so as not to compromise the effectiveness of the diet.

- Meal Planning: Good meal planning is critical to successfully implementing the HCG diet protocol. Plan your meals in advance and make sure you include enough protein, vegetables and fruits in your meals. Pay attention to portion sizes and stick to the recommended amounts of foods allowed.
- Water intake: Drink plenty of water during phase 2 of the HCG diet. Good hydration helps keep your body hydrated, boost metabolism and reduce hunger pangs. Drink at least 8 glasses of water per day and add sugar-free drinks, herbal teas or unsweetened fruit juices as needed.
- Exercise: Although Phase 2 of the HCG diet involves a calorie-restricted diet, moderate exercise is allowed. Add light physical activities such as walking, yoga or stretching into your daily routine. However, always consult

a doctor or qualified trainer before starting a new exercise routine.

Phase 2 of the HCG diet is built on the basis of the HCG diet protocol, which is designed to ensure success. You can lay the groundwork for successful weight loss by taking HCG on a daily basis, adhering to the calorie-restricted diet in a strict manner, selecting the foods that are permitted, engaging in good meal planning, ensuring that you drink enough water, and engaging in appropriate physical activity.

You should make sure that you carefully follow the regimen for the HCG diet, and if you have any doubts or concerns, you should seek the advice of knowledgeable professionals. With the fact that every body is different, it is possible that there are special adaptations that are suitable for you. You can effectively navigate phase 2 of the HCG diet and continue on your journey to effective weight loss if you properly execute the protocol and follow it to the letter.

Ready to put the HCG diet protocol into action and achieve optimal results? Then, let's go on to the following section, where we will delve deeper into the specifics of Phase 2, and prepare ready for the subsequent phases!

4.4 Foods allowed during phase 2

In this section we will look at the foods that are allowed during phase 2 of the HCG diet. It is important to include these foods in your diet to ensure a balanced and calorie-controlled meal plan. Here are some of the foods that are allowed:

- Lean meat: Choose lean meats such as chicken breast, turkey breast, lean beef or lean pork. Remove visible fat before cooking and prepare the meat by roasting, grilling or steaming.
- Fish and seafood: Fish varieties such as cod, salmon, tuna and sole are allowed. You can also enjoy seafood such as shrimp, mussels or crab. Be sure to prepare them gently by grilling, steaming or poaching them.
- Vegetables: There are a variety of vegetables that you can eat during phase 2 of the HCG diet. These include spinach, lettuce, cucumbers, celery, tomatoes, asparagus, broccoli, cabbage, zucchini and peppers. Prepare them

fresh or steam them lightly to preserve their nutrients.

- Fruits: Some fruits are allowed during phase 2 of the HCG diet. These include apples, oranges, grapefruits, strawberries, raspberries and blueberries. Enjoy them as a snack or add them to your salad or yogurt.
- Eggs: Eggs are a good source of protein and can be consumed during phase 2 of the HCG diet. Cook them hard or prepare scrambled eggs or omelets without extra fat.
- Spices and herbs: Use spices and herbs to add flavor to your meals. Salt, pepper, garlic, basil, parsley, oregano and lemon juice are some options you can use.
- Liquids: In addition to water, you can also consume herbal teas, unsweetened teas, black coffee and sugar-free lemonade or fruit juices in moderation during phase 2 of the HCG diet.

You should be sure to keep track of the sizes of your portions and adhere to the recommended amounts of meals that you are permitted to consume. Be sure to take care when preparing foods so that you do not add any additional calories or fat. If you plan and prepare your meals well, you will be able to produce a variety of delicious meals that are within the parameters of the items that are permitted.

For the purpose of planning your meals throughout phase 2 of the HCG diet, you can use this list as a guide. To cater to your own preferences, you can experiment with a variety of different combinations and recipes. Keep in mind that phase 2 is a phase that restricts calories, and in order to achieve the best possible results, you should avoid meals that are not on the list.

During the second phase of the HCG diet, are you prepared to include the specific items that are permitted in your meals? Following, let's move on to the next section, where we will go deeper into the specifics of phase 2, and prepare ready for the subsequent steps!

4.5 Recipes and meal plans for phase 2

As we go on to the next phase of the HCG diet, we will examine the meals and meal plans that are being offered. These recipes and meal plans will assist you in transforming the foods that are permitted into meals that are both inventive and delicious. This is a selection of examples:

Breakfast:

- Scrambled eggs with spinach: Prepare a portion of scrambled eggs with two eggs and add fresh spinach. Season it with salt, pepper and other spices to taste.
- Yogurt with berries: Take a serving of low-fat yogurt and add fresh berries like strawberries or blueberries. You can also use a few drops of liquid stevia for extra sweetness.

Lunch:

- Grilled chicken with vegetables: grill a piece of lean chicken breast fillet and serve it with steamed vegetables such as broccoli, bell bell pepper and zucchini.
- Shrimp salad: Prepare a salad of fresh lettuce leaves, cooked shrimp, cucumbers and tomatoes. Season it with lemon juice and spices of your choice.

Dinner:

- Steamed fish with vegetables: Steam a portion of cod fillet and serve it with steamed vegetables such as asparagus and celery. Season it with herbs and a little lemon juice.
- Beef vegetable stir-fry: Fry lean beef together with vegetables such as bell peppers, zucchini and cabbage. Season it with soy sauce and spices to taste.

Snacks:

Slices of apple or orange that have been sprinkled with cinnamon: To make this dish, slice an apple or orange into thin pieces and then sprinkle them with a slight amount of cinnamon. This is a delectable snack that will leave you feeling full and content.

A low-fat yogurt dip is served alongside vegetable sticks, which are made by slicing fresh veggies like cucumbers, celery, or peppers into sticks and then serving them with the dip.

Keep in mind that throughout phase 2 of the HCG diet, you need to exercise control over the size of your portions. When trying to lose weight, it is important to adhere to the foods that are permitted and the amounts that are recommended. If you want to produce more creative dishes that are still within the parameters of the HCG diet program, you can also try your own individual variants of these recipes.

A weekly meal plan is another option that you may use to assist you in the process of meal planning. You will be able to plan ahead and ensure that you have all of the necessary materials on hand if you employ this method. To ensure that you are getting all of the nutrients that you require, you should plan your meals so that they are both diverse and balanced.

We have high hopes that the following meal plans and dish ideas will provide you with a solid foundation for the second phase of the HCG diet. If you want to make the process of losing weight more fun, try out different flavors and experiment with the foods that are considered acceptable. We will continue our discussion of Phase 2 in the following part, during which we will also provide you with further suggestions and guidance on how to successfully navigate this phase.

4.6 Dealing with hunger and deprivation during phase 2

During the second phase of the HCG diet, we will discuss how you can manage feelings of hunger and deprivation. In this section, we will look at this topic. The intake of calories is highly restricted during this phase, which can make it difficult to deal with, but there are ways to properly manage this complication. I have some advice for you:

- Drink enough water: Often hunger pangs are mistaken for thirst. Make sure you drink enough water to keep your body hydrated. This can help reduce feelings of hunger. Drink small sips of water regularly throughout the day.
- Stick to the meal plan you've been given: A structured meal plan can help you plan your meals in advance and ensure that you eat regularly. This helps minimize hunger pangs. Stick to the recommended portion sizes and allowed foods for best results.

- Use distraction techniques: Distract yourself from hunger pangs by engaging in other activities. Go for a walk, read a book, listen to music, or engage in hobbies you enjoy. Distraction can help take the focus away from food.
- Focus on nutrient-rich foods: Choose foods that fill you up longer and are rich in nutrients. Focus on lean protein sources like chicken breast, fish and eggs, as well as fiber-rich vegetables. These foods can help increase feelings of fullness.
- Use spices and herbs: Spices and herbs can enhance the flavor of meals and help reduce hunger. Experiment with different spices such as garlic, onions, peppers, cinnamon and ginger to vary the flavor of your meals.
- Set realistic expectations: During Phase 2 of the HCG diet, you will likely feel some degree of deprivation. It's important to have realistic expectations and focus on the long-term benefits of weight loss. Keep your goal in mind and stay motivated.
- Seek support: Share your experiences with others who are also on the HCG diet or who want to support you. Talking with like-

minded people can help you overcome challenges and celebrate successes.

During the second phase of the HCG diet, it is not uncommon to experience feelings of hunger and deprivation. You should keep in mind that this period is just temporary and is an essential component of the process that will lead you to achieve your weight loss goals. To successfully deal with hunger and deprivation, it is important to maintain your focus, maintain a positive attitude, and apply these strategies.

As we move on to the following section, we will discuss the subsequent phase of the HCG diet. Stay tuned, and let's continue our adventure together to achieve your goal of losing weight in an effective manner!

Chapter 5: Phase 3 - The stabilization phase

5.1 Purpose and importance of the stabilization phase

We are now moving on to the third phase, which is the phase of stabilization. Within the scope of this chapter, we shall investigate the significance of this phase as well as its goal in greater detail.

Because it serves to stabilize your acquired weight following the phase in which you strictly controlled your calorie intake, the stabilization phase is an extremely important phase because it helps you to keep your weight over the long term. One of the objectives of this phase is to give your body the opportunity to adjust to the new weight and to create a metabolism that is more sustainable. You can succeed over the long term and steer clear of the yo-yo effect if you approach this phase in the right way.

You will progressively reintroduce more foods during the stabilization phase, but you will continue to adhere to certain criteria throughout this process. Establishing good eating habits and achieving a balance between your meals are the primary focuses of this program. While we are at this phase, the following are some crucial considerations to keep in mind:

- Calorie Control: Although you will be consuming more food during this phase, it is important to continue to have proper calorie control. Make sure you don't overeat and that your calorie intake is what your body needs to maintain your new weight.

- Introducing new foods: In the stabilization phase, you can gradually introduce new foods, but pay attention to how your body reacts to them. Add new foods gradually and watch for weight fluctuations or adverse reactions. Make adjustments as necessary to maintain balance.

- Balanced diet: Make sure your meals are balanced and varied. Incorporate a variety of foods that are rich in nutrients, such as fruits, vegetables, lean protein and healthy fats. A balanced diet is key to providing your body with the nutrients it needs and maintaining a healthy weight.

- Watching your weight: During the stabilization phase, it is important to keep an eye on your weight. Weigh yourself regularly and note your progress. If you notice your weight fluctuating or increasing significantly, go back to the guidelines from the previous phase to stabilize your weight.

- Conscious eating and eating behavior: Use the stabilization phase to practice conscious eating and observe your eating behavior. Pay attention to hunger and satiety signals, avoid emotional eating, and find a healthy approach to food. Learn to listen to your body and treat it with respect.

It is during the stabilization period that you will have the opportunity to consolidate the weight loss that you have just accomplished and to continue leading a healthy lifestyle. Make use of this phase to make adjustments to your lifestyle and food that will last for a long time. On the road to long-term success and weight loss that is sustainable, this is a significant step that must be taken.

In the following chapter, we will discuss the maintenance phase of the HCG diet, which is the fifth and last phase of the diet. Stay tuned, and let's keep working together to ensure that you continue to achieve success!

5.2 Guidelines and strategies for phase 3

I would want to offer my congratulations on successfully finishing the phase of tight calorie restriction
and moving on to the phase of stabilization. For the
purpose of successfully managing this phase and
achieving long-term success with weight loss, I will
share with you some crucial suggestions and ideas in
this part.

- Maintain calorie control: Although you will
  eat more foods during the stabilization
  phase, it is important to continue to have adequate calorie control to maintain your new
  weight. Make sure you don't overeat and
  stick to the recommended portion sizes.
- Gradual introduction of new foods: In this
  phase, you can gradually introduce new
  foods. However, it is important to do this
  gradually and observe your reactions. Add a
  new food group and wait a few days to see
  how your body reacts. If there is weight gain
  or other undesirable effects, reduce the
  amount or omit the food for now.

- Focus on healthy, balanced eating: The stabilization phase is a good opportunity to establish a healthy, balanced diet. Make sure your meals are rich in nutrients and contain a balanced mix of protein, vegetables, fruits and healthy fats. Avoid processed foods, sugary snacks and unhealthy fats.
- Continue to follow the HCG diet principles: Although you have more flexibility in the stabilization phase, you should continue to follow the basic principles of the HCG diet. Avoid foods high in sugar and carbohydrates, alcoholic beverages and fatty foods. Stick to the list of allowed foods and follow the portion sizes.
- Maintain an active lifestyle: It is important to remain active during the stabilization phase. Continued physical activity not only helps with weight maintenance, but also contributes to overall health and fitness. Find a form of exercise that you enjoy and incorporate it into your daily routine.

Check your weight on a regular basis: It is essential to continue checking your weight on a frequent basis when you are in the stability period. Be on the lookout for significant shifts in your weight pattern. If your weight is more than 900 grams higher than what you have attained, you should take action to get back to the weight that you have set as your goal. You can also make use of the strategies that you successfully used in the phase before this one.

As you progress through the stability phase, you will have the opportunity to solidify your success and achieve weight loss that is sustainable over time. Establishing good eating habits and maintaining your weight over the long term can be accomplished by adhering to these principles and utilizing the solutions. In order to realize the benefits of your efforts and live a life that is both healthier and more satisfying, you will need to adopt a method that is both aware and disciplined.

Within the following chapter, we will discuss the maintenance phase of the HCG diet, which is the final step of the diet. At that location, we will talk about ways in which you can sustainably maintain your weight and maintain a healthy lifestyle while doing so. So keep your motivation up, and let's keep working together to ensure that you achieve success!

5.3 Introduction of new food groups

During the phase of the HCG diet known as "stabilization," it is time to gradually incorporate additional food groups into your diet. Due to this, you will be able to broaden your food choices and continue to consume a diet that is both varied and balanced. However, it is essential to do this in a progressive manner in order to guarantee that your body will react positively and that you will be able to maintain a steady weight.

During this phase, you may choose to provide the following new food groups to your customers:

- Whole grain products: You can slowly introduce whole grain products like whole wheat bread, whole wheat pasta, oatmeal and brown rice. These provide fiber and nutrients and are a healthy addition to your diet. Be sure to keep portion sizes in mind and don't overload yourself with these foods.
- Dairy products: You can now introduce low-fat dairy products like yogurt, cottage cheese and low-fat cheeses. These provide high-quality protein and calcium, which is important for bone health. Make sure you

choose the low-fat varieties and limit your consumption of high-fat dairy products.

- Fruit varieties: During the stabilization phase, you can expand your selection of fruits. Gradually add new fruits to increase variety and boost your intake of vitamins and antioxidants. However, be sure to continue to eat high-sugar fruits like bananas and grapes in moderation.

- Vegetables: You can now enjoy a wider variety of vegetables. Add new varieties to add variety to your meals and get different nutrients. Make sure you continue to avoid starchy vegetables like potatoes and corn and focus on non-starchy vegetables like green leafy vegetables, cucumbers, tomatoes and peppers.

- Healthy fats: In the stabilization phase, you can include healthy fats in your diet. These include avocado, nuts, seeds and healthy vegetable oils like olive oil and coconut oil. These fats provide important nutrients and support healthy heart function. However, be sure to keep track of quantities, as fats have a high caloric density.

As you introduce new food categories into your diet, it is essential to pay attention to how your body reacts to these changes. Pay attention to any indications of weight gain, a feeling of bloating, or any other unfavorable symptoms. Reduce the amount of particular food groups or leave them out entirely for the time being if you find that they are having a detrimental impact on your health.

Make use of this phase to broaden the variety of foods you consume and to locate a healthy balance. You may get the benefits of a diversified diet by trying out different recipes and experimenting with them. If you adhere to the instructions and tactics that are presented throughout this phase, you will be able to accomplish your weight loss objectives and keep a healthy weight for the duration of the next phase.

In the following chapter, we will discuss the maintenance phase of the HCG diet, which refers to the ultimate portion of the program. In that section, we will talk about how you can keep your weight at the level you have achieved over the long term while also maintaining a healthy lifestyle. Stay tuned, and let's keep working together to ensure that you continue to achieve success!

5.4 Maintaining the achieved weight

Congratulations! You have been successful in reaching the weight that you desired. Nevertheless, the journey is not yet complete. When you are in the stability phase, your primary focus should be on leading a healthy lifestyle and preserving the weight that you have achieved over an extended period of time. To assist you in maintaining your weight loss, the following are some essential principles and strategies:

- Continuity in eating habits: It's important to maintain the healthy eating habits you developed while on the HCG diet. Continue to eat balanced meals that are rich in lean protein, fresh vegetables, fruits and healthy fats. Avoid falling back into old eating habits and stay consistent with a healthy diet.
- Keeping an eye on portions: During the stabilization phase, it is critical to keep an eye on portion sizes. Overeating can lead to weight gain. Continue to use a kitchen scale

or visual references to estimate proper portion sizes and control your caloric intake.

- Regular Physical Activity: Keep up your physical activity to boost your metabolism and support your energy levels. Engage in regular exercise, whether it's aerobics, strength training or other activities you enjoy. Stay active and find ways to incorporate exercise into your daily routine.
- Awareness of your body reactions: Pay attention to your body's reactions when you try new foods or activities. Everyone's body reacts differently, so it's important to recognize what works for you personally and what doesn't. Listen to your sense of satiety and pay attention to how different foods affect your well-being.
- Avoid stress: Stress can have a negative impact on your weight and health. Find ways to reduce stress, whether through meditation, relaxation techniques or activities you enjoy. A balanced and stress-free life will support your weight management goals.
- Regular checkups and support: Schedule regular checkups with your doctor or dietitian to monitor your progress and get further support. They can help you overcome

potential challenges and offer solutions to maintain your weight long-term.

If you adhere to these principles and tactics and continue to live a mindful lifestyle, you will be able to keep the weight that you have achieved and continue to feel healthy and energized over the long term. In the event that you experience failures, do not allow yourself to become disheartened. Maintain your concentration, wait patiently, and keep in mind that you have already achieved success. In order to live a life that is both healthy and rewarding, you have the capacity to maintain control of your weight.

5.5 Transition to the maintenance phase

Congratulations! As a result of your successful completion of the Stabilization Phase, you are now prepared to move on to the Maintenance Phase. In this part of the article, we will talk about how to successfully plan for and carry out the Maintenance Phase. Listed below are some essential actions that should be kept in mind:

- Set a schedule: Consider a time frame for the maintenance phase. It is recommended to spend at least three weeks in this phase to give your body time to adjust to the weight you have achieved and maintain a stable metabolism.
- Gradual introduction of new foods: During the maintenance phase, you can gradually introduce new foods into your diet. It is important to do this gradually and in a controlled way to observe possible effects on your weight and well-being. Start with foods that were avoided during the HCG diet and watch how your body reacts to them.
- Watching your weight: Continue to keep an eye on your weight as you introduce new foods. It can be helpful to do regular weight and measure checks to make sure you are maintaining the weight you have reached. If you notice that your weight is increasing, you can make appropriate adjustments to your diet.
- Portions and calorie control: Even in the maintenance phase, it is important to keep track of portion sizes and control calorie intake. Make sure you continue to eat balanced

meals and don't let the discipline of the previous phases distract you.

- Continuing physical activity: Stay active! Regular physical activity is important even in the maintenance phase to keep your metabolism up and support a healthy weight. Find activities you enjoy and incorporate exercise into your daily routine.
- Develop long-term strategies: Use the maintenance phase to develop long-term strategies for healthy weight management. Think about what foods and habits work best for you to control your weight. Set realistic goals and find a healthy and sustainable way to maintain the weight you achieve.

It is essential to keep in mind that the phase of maintenance is an essential component of your quest to lose weight. You will be able to maintain a healthy lifestyle and consolidate the results of the previous phases throughout the course of a longer period of time with its assistance. Maintain your concentration, exercise patience, and have faith in your capacity to do what you set out to do. You have already demonstrated that you are capable of bringing about significant changes in your life when you take action.

Have fun during the maintenance phase, and be happy with your accomplishments!

Chapter 6: Phase 4 - The maintenance phase

6.1 The importance of the maintenance phase

Congratulations! The HCG diet has been successfully completed, and you have achieved the weight that you had set for yourself. The next step, which is the maintenance phase, is a crucial one since it is during this period that you will learn how to keep your new weight and maintain a healthy lifestyle. In this section, we will conduct a more in-depth examination of the significance of the maintenance phase, as well as provide you with the techniques and recommendations that you require in order to achieve success over the course of time.

Because of the so-called yo-yo effect, which occurs when weight is quickly recovered following a diet, the maintenance phase is extremely important in order to stabilize the results that you have achieved. The goal of this phase is to provide your body with the necessary time to adjust to the new weight and to keep your metabolism stable. In the maintenance phase, the following are some key elements to consider:

- Set a time frame: Plan at least three weeks for the maintenance phase to give your body enough time to stabilize. Some people even choose to continue this phase longer to ensure that their weight remains stable. It is important to be patient and realize that the maintenance phase is an important part of the process.
- Monitoring your weight: Even in the maintenance phase, it is advisable to perform regular weight checks to ensure that you maintain the weight you have reached. It is normal for weight to fluctuate slightly, but make sure you stay within a certain range. If you notice the weight shifting up or down, you can make adjustments accordingly.
- Maintain a healthy diet: The maintenance phase is not a return to old eating habits. It is important to maintain the healthy diet you practiced during the HCG diet. Continue to eat a balanced diet with plenty of fresh vegetables, lean protein and healthy fats. Avoid excessive consumption of sugar, refined carbohydrates and processed foods.
- Portion control and conscious eating: Watch portion sizes and practice conscious eating.

Listen to your body and eat only when you are truly hungry. Avoid eating for emotional reasons or letting outside influences guide you. Choose high quality foods that provide your body with nutrients and fill you up.

- Continue physical activity: Stay active and incorporate regular exercise into your daily routine. Physical activity not only supports weight maintenance, but also has many other health benefits. Find activities that you enjoy and can maintain long-term. Whether it's walking, yoga, strength training or other sports, find what suits you.
- Continuous self-reflection: The maintenance phase offers you the opportunity to get to know yourself better and to rethink your long-term goals. Ask yourself what is important to you and how you can integrate a healthy lifestyle permanently. Set realistic goals and find ways to develop yourself and improve your well-being.

It is a joyful period when you are able to reap the results of your hard work and permanently lock in your new weight. This phase is known as the maintenance phase. Take use of this phase to strengthen the behaviors you've just gained, continue your education, and adjust to a lifestyle that is more healthy and is more balanced. Have faith in yourself and your capacity to achieve success over the course of time. You are deserving of a life that is full of joy and good health.

6.2 Guidelines and strategies for the maintenance phase

In this area, we will give you with vital suggestions and ideas to guarantee that you are able to keep the weight that you have reached over the long term and live a life that is healthy and balanced. In order to assist you in effectively navigating the maintenance period, the following recommendations provide assistance:

- Stay consistent with healthy eating: Even in the maintenance phase, it is important to maintain a healthy diet. Continue to focus on fresh vegetables, lean protein, whole grains and healthy fats. Avoid overly processed foods, sugary snacks and soft drinks.

Introduce a balanced meal plan that provides adequate nutrients and fills you up.

- Maintain portion control: Continue to watch the size of your meals and practice conscious eating. Avoid overeating and make sure you only eat as much as your body needs. Listen to your body's signals and stop when you feel full. A good way to keep track of portion sizes is to use smaller plates and bowls.

- Incorporate regular exercise: Stay active and incorporate regular physical activity into your daily routine. Choose activities that you enjoy and can maintain long-term. Whether it's walking, biking, dancing, swimming or yoga, find a form of exercise that suits you and that you can do regularly. Exercise will not only help you maintain your weight, but it will also increase your energy levels and improve your overall well-being.

- Continuous self-reflection: Use the maintenance phase to get to know yourself better and to rethink your relationship with food and body weight. Reflect regularly on your progress, goals and challenges. Find ways to motivate yourself and reinforce positive

habits. Be patient with yourself and accept
that there may be normal ups and downs.
Stay focused on your long-term goals and
continually work to find a healthy balance.

- Seek support: It can be helpful to seek support in the form of friends, family or a community who share similar goals. Sharing, motivation and mutual support can help navigate through challenges and maintain the weight you've achieved. Look for online forums, social media groups or local meetups to connect with like-minded people.

Make sure you are adaptable and pay attention to your health concerns: There is no "one-size-fits-all" option for the maintenance phase because every body is different and can be treated differently. Take the time to pay attention to what your body is telling you, and be willing to make changes if something isn't functioning properly. Experiment with a variety of methods and see which one works best for you. Always be sure to pay attention to your health and, if required, seek the assistance of a professional who can assist you in achieving your objectives.

When it comes to ensuring that the results of the HCG diet are maintained over the long term, the maintenance phase is the most important step. You will be able to keep your weight at a healthy level and continue to feel fantastic if you adhere to these rules and tactics and live a life that is healthy and balanced. Be proud of your accomplishments, and keep your attention on leading a life that is both healthy and pleasant. You are deserving of it!

6.3 Long-term weight control after the HCG diet

Currently, you are interested in ensuring that you are able to keep a healthy weight for an extended period of time. As we move on with the HCG diet, we will now move on to the next section, where we will address crucial techniques and tips for long-term weight control.

- Stick to healthy eating habits: The HCG diet has helped you change your eating habits and focus on healthy foods. Stick to it and incorporate a balanced diet rich in vegetables, lean protein, whole grains and healthy fats. Avoid overly processed foods and sugary snacks. Focus on a sustainable diet that gives you enough nutrients and keeps you full.

- Track your weight regularly: Monitor your weight regularly to develop an awareness of how your body is behaving. It is important to note that natural weight fluctuations are normal. Avoid weighing yourself daily, as this can lead to Unnecessary Stress. Choose a specific day of the week and time to weigh yourself and keep track of progress.

- Stay active: Regular physical activity is an essential part of long-term weight control. Find an activity that you enjoy and can incorporate into your daily routine. Whether it's walking, running, swimming, strength training or yoga, find a form of exercise that you enjoy and can do regularly. Exercise not only helps with weight maintenance, but it also helps improve your health and mood.

- Set realistic goals: Set realistic and achievable goals for your long-term weight control. It's important not to set unrealistic expectations for yourself. The focus should be on a healthy lifestyle and well-being, not just the number on the scale. Take time to celebrate your successes and reward yourself in other ways that have nothing to do with food.

- Stick to your lessons from the HCG diet: The HCG diet has taught you important lessons about nutrition and self-control. Use these experiences and insights to continue eating healthy and living mindfully. Remember the positive effects you experienced during the diet and let them motivate you to maintain your healthy habits.
- Seek support: It can be helpful to seek support from friends, family or other people who have similar goals. Interact with them, share your experiences and find mutual support. Together, you can motivate each other and work together toward your long-term goals.

On the path to long-term weight control, the HCG diet is one step along the way; but, in order to maintain weight control over the long term, sustained effort and adjustments in lifestyle are required. You can keep your weight under control and live a life that is both healthy and joyful if you employ the appropriate tactics and maintain a good mindset. Keep your attention on the task at hand, have patience with yourself, and have faith that you are in charge of your weight. You have the potential to do what you set out to do in the long run!

6.4 Maintain healthy eating habits

At this point in the HCG diet, you have reached the maintenance phase, which is all about ensuring that your healthy eating habits are maintained for the long term. It is essential that you complete this phase in order to keep the weight that you have attained and to make a change in your lifestyle that is lasting. In order to assist you in maintaining good eating habits, the following tips and practices are provided:

- Continue to choose healthy foods: Even after the HCG diet, it is important to continue to choose healthy foods. Focus on a balanced diet rich in fruits, vegetables, lean protein, whole grains and healthy fats. Avoid overly processed foods, sugary snacks and fast food. Go for fresh, natural ingredients and prepare your own meals to have full control over your diet.
- Pay attention to portion control: Keep an awareness of portion sizes and learn to eat intuitively. Listen to your body and stop when you feel full. Avoid overeating and be

mindful when eating. Take time to enjoy your meals and consciously notice the flavors. If you feel you need a smaller portion, don't hesitate to adjust.

- Maintain a regular meal structure: Stick to a regular meal structure and try to eat meals at the same time. This helps maintain stable blood sugar levels and avoid cravings. Plan your meals in advance and prepare healthy snacks to keep you energized throughout the day.

- Listen to your body: Be mindful and listen to your body's needs. Pay attention to hunger and fullness signals and respond accordingly. If you're feeling stressed or emotional, try to find alternative ways to cope instead of reaching for food. Find healthy coping strategies such as meditation, exercise, or sharing with friends.

- Reward yourself in other ways: Reward yourself in ways other than food. Find alternative rewards that motivate you and bring you joy. These can be activities you enjoy, such as a trip to nature, a new book, a relaxing bath, or time with friends and family.

Learn that rewards don't always have to involve food.

- Continue to track your progress: Set long-term goals and continue to track your progress. Keep a journal of your diet and activities to keep track of your habits. This can help keep you accountable and make adjustments when necessary.

When it comes to advancement and stability, the maintenance phase is the time to be. Keep your attention on the task at hand, commit to adopting healthy eating habits, and have faith that you possess the resources necessary to keep the weight you've attained for the long term. You will arrive at a life that is both healthier and happier as a result of this adventure.

6.5 Dealing with relapses and setbacks

While you are working toward your goals of losing weight and achieving your objectives, there will be times when you may experience relapses or setbacks. Understand that this is a natural part of the process and that it should not be considered a failure. This is a crucial point to keep in sight. In order to deal with relapses and setbacks, the following strategies might be utilized:

- Understand the reason for the relapse: Honestly analyze the reasons for the relapse. Was it an emotional trigger, stress, or a particular event? By identifying the causes, you can better understand why you relapsed and respond accordingly.
- Avoid blaming yourself: Don't blame yourself. Everyone has a bad day or a difficult period. Accept the setback as part of the process and allow yourself to learn from it. Be kind and compassionate to yourself.
- Learn from the relapse: Use the relapse as an opportunity to reflect and grow. Ask yourself what you learned from the situation and what actions you can take to better handle similar situations in the future. Realize that every setback can be a lesson that makes you stronger.
- Set realistic goals: Review your goals and make sure they are realistic and achievable. Sometimes too high expectations can lead to frustration and disappointment, which paves

the way for setbacks. Set small goals that you
can achieve step by step, and celebrate any
progress you make.

- Seek support: Don't let yourself be alone
  with your setbacks. Seek support from
  friends, family or a support group. Share
  your challenges and successes and let others
  motivate you. Together, you can encourage
  and support each other to get back on track.

- Stay positive and keep going: Don't use relapse as an excuse to give up. Stay positive
  and remind yourself that you have already
  made a lot of progress. Focus on what you
  have already accomplished and be proud of
  yourself. Don't let a setback discourage you,
  but see it as an opportunity to come back
  even stronger.

On the HCG diet, you will experience a trip that may
be full of both highs and lows. Keeping a positive attitude in the face of failure is of the utmost importance. Keep your attention on your long-term objective of losing weight in a way that is both healthy
and sustainable, and learn from them and improve
as a result of them. Your resilience allows you to recover quickly from any failure and carry on with
your life in a successful manner. You should have

faith in yourself and remain steadfast in your pursuit
of a life that is both healthy and fulfilling.

Chapter 7: HCG diet and physical activity

7.1 The role of exercise during the HCG diet

During the HCG diet, exercise and other forms of physical activity continue to play a vital role. On the other hand, regular exercise can bring extra benefits and promote the process of weight loss, even though the diet itself is intended to minimize the number of calories consumed. Exercising is essential during the HCG diet for a number of reasons, including the following:

- Metabolism support: You can boost your metabolism through physical activity. Regular exercise increases energy expenditure and helps burn excess calories. This can accelerate weight loss and lead to more effective fat burning.
- Maintaining muscle mass: During the HCG diet, the goal is to lose fat, not muscle mass. You can strengthen and maintain your muscles through targeted exercise, especially strength training. This is important to keep the body toned and defined and to promote a healthy body composition.

- Improving well-being: Exercise not only has positive effects on the body, but also on mental and emotional health. Regular physical activity can reduce stress, improve mood and enhance overall well-being. During the HCG diet, which can be fraught with challenges and changes, exercise can serve as a balance and help relieve stress.

- Maintaining an active lifestyle: The HCG diet is not a short-term approach to weight loss, but is designed to lead to long-term changes. By incorporating exercise into your daily routine, you'll develop an active lifestyle that can be maintained even after the diet is complete. Regular physical activity supports long-term weight control and can help you feel fit, energetic and healthy.

When selecting activities that are suitable for the HCG diet, it is essential to take into consideration the individual's specific requirements and constraints. You have the option of selecting from a variety of options for physical activity, including swimming, yoga, weight training, and aerobics. Discover a pastime that you take pleasure in and that you can easily fit into your everyday routine.

In addition to this, it is essential to pay attention to your body and make sure you get enough rest. The HCG diet might be difficult to follow, and it is essential to allow your body sufficient time to recuperate after each meal.

During the HCG diet, it is important to keep in mind that physical activity is not required, but rather a supplement that can boost your results and promote your overall well-being. Pay attention to what your body is telling you, choose the appropriate degree of activity for you, and take pleasure in the positive effects that exercise has on both your physical and mental health.

7.2 Suitable forms of physical activity

During the HCG diet, there are many different kinds of physical activity that may be easily incorporated into the diet plan. These activities can have a great impact on both the weight reduction and the health of the individual. During your time on the HCG diet, you might want to consider participating in the following activities:

- Walking: Walking is an easy and accessible form of physical activity that you can do anywhere, anytime. Whether you're walking outside or running on a treadmill at the gym, regular walking can boost your metabolism and support weight loss.
- Cycling: Cycling is a great way to burn calories while improving your endurance. You can ride a bike outdoors or take indoor spinning classes. Cycling is easy on the joints and is a great way to increase your physical activity.
- Swimming: Swimming is an excellent full-body exercise that strengthens muscles and tones the body. It is also an activity that is easy on the joints, especially for people who struggle with joint problems. Swimming can boost metabolism and aid weight loss.
- Strength training: Strength training is an important addition to physical activity during the HCG diet. By strengthening your

muscles, you help increase metabolism and keep your body toned and defined. You can work with weights, use resistance bands, or do bodyweight exercises like push-ups and squats.

- Yoga or Pilates: These forms of holistic exercise can be beneficial during the HCG diet, as they not only provide physical activity, but also promote relaxation and stress reduction. Yoga and Pilates can help improve flexibility, strength and body awareness.

It should be emphasized that any kind of physical activity should be tailored to the specific needs of the individual. Adapt the level of intensity and duration of your activities to your needs and the state of your physical condition by paying attention to your body. To prevent damage, begin cautiously and gradually increase your intensity.

For the purpose of ensuring that you are performing the exercises appropriately and getting the most out of your physical activity, it is also a good idea to collaborate with a certified personal trainer or fitness expert.

During the HCG diet, it is important to keep in mind that physical activity is really a supplement and not the primary goal. For maximum results, it is recommended that you combine physical activity with a nutritious diet and other components of the HCG diet program. Take pleasure in the many activities, discover the pleasure in physical activity, and allow it to become an essential component of your healthy lifestyle.

7.3 Training tips during the different phases of the HCG diet

When following the HCG diet, it is essential to engage in the appropriate physical activity in order to make the most of the potential benefits of the diet and to attain the outcomes that are wanted. While you are going through the various stages of the HCG diet, here are some helpful fitness tips that you can take into consideration:

Phase 1: Loading or preparation phase

- In this phase, the focus is on replenishing the body's energy stores. It is therefore not necessary to perform intensive training.
- You can incorporate lighter activities like walking, gentle yoga or stretching into your daily routine.
- The goal is to stay active and prepare your body for the phases ahead.

Phase 2: Strictly calorie restricted phase

- During this phase, the calorie deficit is high, so it is important to adjust training to avoid overloading the body.
- Focus on light to moderate aerobic activities like walking, biking or swimming.
- Avoid intense cardio workouts or longer workouts because your body has less energy available during the calorie-restricted phase.

Phase 3: Stabilization phase

- In this phase you have more freedom in choosing your training activities.
- You can gradually increase your physical activity and incorporate more intense workouts like strength training or HIIT training into your workouts.
- The goal is to maintain your muscle mass, boost metabolism and maintain a healthy body composition.

Phase 4: Maintenance phase

- In this phase you can design your training according to your preferences and goals.
- You can choose a combination of strength training, cardio and flexibility exercises to keep your body fit and healthy.
- Experiment with different workouts and find out what you enjoy and fits your lifestyle.

In spite of the fact that you are now in a cycle, it is of the utmost importance to pay attention to your body and to avoid overworking it. You should begin with an adequate level of intensity and gradually raise it as you move through the exercise. In order to avoid getting wounded, it is essential to pay attention to your technique and to perform the exercises in the correct manner.

If you are unsure of what you want to accomplish with your training or if you have specific goals in mind, it is my recommended that you seek the guidance of a licensed personal trainer or fitness professional. They are able to provide assistance in the process of establishing a specialized training program that is suited to your particular requirements and goals.

Keeping in mind that the HCG diet is not the primary focus, but rather the one that complements it, is an essential point to bear in mind. When paired with other aspects of the HCG diet program, like as a nutritious food, adequate rest, and other elements, it has the potential to result in success over the long term. Exercise should be something you look forward to, it should be a part of your healthy lifestyle, and you should be happy that you are making progress toward your goal of losing weight.

7.4 The importance of strength training

In addition to being an essential part of a holistic fitness regimen, strength training is also an essential component of maintaining a healthy weight while following the HCG diet. You are going to gain an understanding of the significance of strength training as well as the ways in which you can include it into your path to lose weight.

- Building muscle mass: Strength training is the key to building and maintaining muscle mass. During the HCG diet, a calorie-restricted diet can cause the body to lose muscle mass. Through regular strength training, you can counteract this effect and maintain or even build your muscle mass. Muscle tissue has the advantage of burning more energy than fat tissue, which in turn boosts your metabolism and contributes to more effective weight loss.
- Body sculpting: Strength training allows you to shape your body contours and achieve a more toned figure. By targeting specific

muscle groups, you can address your problem areas and make your body look more proportioned. The result is improved body composition and an aesthetically pleasing appearance.

- Strengthening the body: Strength training not only strengthens your muscles, but also your bones, ligaments and tendons. This reduces the risk of injury and improves your overall physical performance. You'll find that you have more strength in everyday life and feel fitter and more energetic overall.
- Increased fat burning: The strength training itself burns calories, but the real benefit is that it increases the afterburn effect. After an intense strength training session, your metabolism remains elevated for hours as the body needs energy to recover and rebuild muscle mass. This leads to increased fat burning, even during rest periods.

To reap the benefits of strength training while on the HCG diet, you should keep a few important points in mind:

- Start with an appropriate training program tailored to your individual needs and goals. A qualified trainer can help you create a customized program.
- Perform exercises correctly and maintain good form to avoid injury. If necessary, seek the guidance of an expert.
- Start with moderate weight and gradually increase to challenge your muscles and progress.
- Incorporate different exercises for different muscle groups to train your body holistically.
- Consider your individual fitness level and adjust your training accordingly. Listen to your body and don't go beyond your limits.

Remember that strength training is a valuable complement to the other aspects of the HCG diet, including diet and doing other activities. It's a way to support your weight loss goals and achieve a healthy, strong and well-shaped body image in the long run.

7.5 Overcoming obstacles and injuries

During the course of your journey to achieve your weight loss objective, you can come into challenges that can present you with challenges and create injury-related setbacks. Identifying these challenges and coming up with solutions to overcome them is an essential step in conquering them. While on the HCG diet, the following are some suggestions that will assist you in overcoming challenges and injuries:

- Stay positive: A positive attitude is the key to overcoming obstacles. Accept that setbacks are normal and view them as opportunities to learn from and come back stronger. Don't let frustration or disappointment discourage you, but stay focused and motivated.
- Listen to your body: Your body is a valuable tool that sends you signals. When you feel pain or injury, it's important to listen to your body and take appropriate action. This may mean adjusting a workout session, taking a break, or seeking professional medical help. Be aware of your limits and don't exceed them to avoid injury.
- Consult experts: If you are facing obstacles or injuries, it is advisable to seek expert advice.

A qualified doctor, physical therapist or trainer can help you plan appropriate treatment and rehabilitation. They can also make recommendations for alternative exercises or adaptations to continue your training.

- Adapt your training: Depending on the type of injury or obstacle, you may need to adjust your workouts or find alternative activities that don't stress you. Talk to an expert about appropriate exercises that won't aggravate your injury but still support your fitness goals. Remember that even a modified activity is better than none at all.

- Use alternative strategies: If you're temporarily limited due to injury or other obstacles, use the time to strengthen other aspects of your weight loss journey. Focus on healthy eating, mental wellness and rest to support your body. Be patient and give yourself the time you need to recover.

You should keep in mind that challenges and injuries are a natural part of the process of losing weight, but you should not let them deter you. With the appropriate mindset, support, and the capacity to adapt, you will be able to triumph over these obstacles and accomplish what you set out to do. Maintain your concentration, have patience with yourself, and resist the want to give up. It is within your ability to triumph over challenges and make improvements to your physical health and fitness.

Chapter 8: HCG diet and possible side effects

8.1 Overview of possible side effects

Some side effects may possibly occur with the HCG diet. It is important to be aware of these potential effects and take appropriate action. Here is a comprehensive overview of possible side effects of the HCG diet:

- Fatigue: Fatigue may occur during the calorie-restricted phases of the HCG diet. This is due to the low calorie content and the body's adaptation to the change in metabolism. It is important to get enough sleep to minimize fatigue.
- Headaches: Some people report headaches during the HCG diet. This may be due to the abrupt elimination of certain foods or the loss of fluids. It is important to drink enough fluids and take pain relievers if necessary.
- Constipation: Due to the change in dietary habits and limited fiber intake, some people may struggle with constipation during the

HCG diet. It is recommended to consume high fiber foods such as vegetables and whole grains and drink enough water to aid in digestion.

- Muscle loss: Since the HCG diet involves a low-calorie diet, there is a possibility that the body will lose muscle mass for energy. To counteract this, it is important to consume enough protein and perform regular physical activities such as strength training.
- Mood swings: Some people may experience mood swings during the HCG diet. This may be due to the hormonal influence of HCG and the low calorie diet. It is important to pay attention to emotional well-being and seek support if necessary.
- Water retention: You may experience temporary water retention during the HCG diet, especially in the first few days. This is a normal reaction of the body to the changes in diet. The water retention should normalize over time.

It is essential to keep in mind that not everyone will suffer each and every one of these adverse effects. Depending on the individual, the consequences could be different. However, it is recommended that you pay attention to the reactions that your own body is experiencing and, if required, seek help and advice from a knowledgeable nutritionist or a medical professional.

Keep in mind that the majority of the signs and symptoms are only transient and should improve over time. In the event that adverse effects continue or become serious, it is essential to seek the counsel of a professional. Monitoring and modifying your food and lifestyle in a comprehensive manner can help reduce the likelihood of experiencing adverse effects and enhance the likelihood of successfully losing weight.

8.2 Dealing with hunger and lack of energy

It is possible that the HCG diet will cause you to experience symptoms of hunger and a lack of energy on occasion. The recognition of these difficulties and the implementation of proper measures to address them are both extremely important. Here are some suggestions that can assist you in controlling your hunger and keeping your energy levels up:

- Drink enough water: Thirst is often confused with hunger. Therefore, drink water regularly to quench your thirst and reduce hunger pangs. Aim to drink at least 2 liters of water per day.
- Keep yourself distracted: Distraction can help overcome hunger pangs. Engage in activities that require your attention, such as walking, reading, listening to music, or talking with friends and family. This can help you think less about food.
- Choose filling foods: Be sure to choose foods that keep you full longer. This includes high-fiber foods like vegetables, whole grains, and high-protein foods like lean meats, fish, eggs, and legumes. These foods help reduce your hunger pangs and keep your energy up.
- Plan meals and snacks in advance: By planning your meals and snacks in advance, you can ensure that you have balanced and nutritious options available. This will help you control hunger and prevent energy deficiencies. Prepare healthy snacks like fruit, vegetable sticks or nuts to have on hand when hunger strikes.
- Eat small meals regularly: Instead of eating large meals, try eating smaller meals

regularly throughout the day. This helps keep blood sugar levels stable and helps control hunger. Plan three main meals and one or two snacks to meet your energy needs.

- Check your calorie intake: Make sure you are eating enough calories to meet your energy needs. The HCG diet involves a calorie-restricted diet, but it is important that you get enough nutrients to support your body. Consult a doctor or nutritionist to make sure you are following the right amount of calories for your individual needs.
- Listen to your body: Pay attention to your body's signals and learn to distinguish between real hunger and emotional hunger. If you're really hungry, eat a balanced meal or a healthy snack. Avoid overeating out of boredom, stress, or other emotional reasons.

By using these strategies, you can reduce hunger pangs and maintain your energy during the HCG diet. It's important to be patient with yourself and focus on giving your body the nutrients it needs to stay healthy and energized.

8.3 Dealing with emotional fluctuations

It is possible that you could experience mood swings while you are on the HCG diet since your body will be adjusting to the changes in your food. It is critical to be aware of these feelings and to employ constructive methods in order to be able to control them. While you are on the HCG diet, here are some suggestions that can assist you in managing your emotional swings:

- Recognize and accept your feelings: Emotional fluctuations are normal and can occur due to changes in caloric intake and hormonal balance. Take time to recognize your feelings and accept them as part of the process.
- Find alternative stress management methods: Instead of comforting yourself with food, look for healthy stress management methods such as meditation, yoga, taking a walk or writing in a journal. These activities can help you relieve stress and manage your emotional swings.
- Build social support: Talk to friends, family members or other people who support you during your HCG diet. Share your feelings

and experiences with them for emotional support. Sometimes just having someone listen and show understanding helps.

- Avoid harsh self-criticism: Be gentle with yourself and avoid criticizing yourself when you are feeling emotional. Remind yourself that these are temporary fluctuations and that you are making progress. Be patient and positive with yourself.
- Get enough sleep: Sleep plays an important role in your emotional stability. Make sure to get enough sleep to give your body the rest it needs. Schedule regular bedtimes and create a relaxing sleep environment.
- Avoid extra stress: Try to avoid extra stress during the HCG diet. Prioritize your tasks and reduce the number of commitments if possible. Create a work-life balance and allow yourself to take breaks and relax.
- Seek professional support: If you feel your emotional swings are excessive or persistent, don't be afraid to seek professional support. A therapist or counselor can help you better understand your emotions and develop healthy coping strategies.

Through the utilization of these tactics, you will be better able to manage emotional swings while on the HCG diet. Take into consideration that every single person is unique and that it is perfectly natural to feel a variety of emotions. You should allow yourself the time and space to accept your sentiments and concentrate on the road that will lead to weight loss that is sustainable.

8.4 Common misconceptions and myths about the HCG diet

The HCG diet has attracted a lot of attention in recent years, which has led to various misconceptions and myths. It is important to clarify these misconceptions in order to gain a better understanding of the HCG diet. Here are some common misconceptions and myths about the HCG diet that should be cleared up:

Myth: HCG is a miracle cure for weight loss.

Truth: HCG alone is not a miracle cure for weight loss. The HCG diet combines a low calorie diet with the use of HCG to aid in weight loss. It is important to understand that the weight loss is primarily due to the low calorie diet.

Myth: HCG diet is dangerous and unhealthy.

Truth: When done correctly and under a doctor's supervision, the HCG diet is usually safe and effective. However, it is important to follow the HCG diet only for the intended period of time and according to the instructions. Always consult a doctor or qualified nutritionist before starting any diet.

Myth: The HCG diet leads to muscle loss.

Truth: Combining HCG with a low-calorie diet encourages the body to use fat reserves as a source of energy instead of breaking down muscle mass. However, it is important to consume sufficient protein during the diet to minimize muscle loss.

Myth: After finishing the HCG diet, the yo-yo effect occurs.

Truth: The yo-yo effect often occurs when returning to old eating habits after a diet. To avoid the yo-yo effect, it is important to gradually and healthily transition to a balanced diet after the HCG diet. The maintenance phase of the HCG diet plays an important role in this.

Myth: The HCG diet is suitable for everyone.

Truth: HCG diet is not suitable for everyone. People with certain health conditions or during pregnancy should avoid the HCG diet. It is important to consult a doctor before starting the diet and make sure that there are no contraindications.

It is important to clear up these misconceptions and myths about the HCG diet to promote proper understanding. The HCG diet can be effective when done correctly, but it is important to follow the guidelines and seek medical advice. Trust sound information and be skeptical of unrealistic promises or unsubstantiated claims.

8.5 Consultation with a doctor before starting the HCG diet

Before you start the HCG diet, it is important to have a thorough medical consultation. A doctor can give you important information and evaluate your suitability for the HCG diet. Here are some reasons why consulting a doctor before starting the HCG diet is important:

- Medical monitoring: A doctor can evaluate your overall health and determine if there are any medical conditions that may militate against following the HCG diet. This is especially important if you already have health problems or are taking medication.
- Customization: Every body is unique, and it is important to customize a diet to your individual needs. A doctor can determine if the HCG diet is right for you and if adjustments need to be made to ensure you get optimal results.
- Safety: A doctor can give you information about potential risks and side effects of the HCG diet. They can inform you about

possible drug interactions and give you instructions on how to follow the diet safely.

- Support and care: A doctor can provide ongoing support during your HCG diet. They can help you monitor your progress, identify any problems and take appropriate action.
- During the medical consultation, you should be honest about your health history, medications and other relevant factors. This way, the doctor can make an informed decision and adapt the HCG diet to your individual needs.

Remember that consulting a doctor before starting the HCG diet is to ensure your health and safety. It is an important step to ensure that you are following the diet in a safe manner and getting maximum benefits from it. Don't hesitate to make an appointment with a qualified doctor to discuss any questions or concerns you have. Together you can decide if the HCG diet is right for you and how best to implement it.

Chapter 9: HCG diet and sustainability

9.1 Long-term effects of the HCG diet

The HCG diet has the potential to be an efficient method for achieving weight loss and improving one's body composition. How about the effects that will last for a long time? Is it possible to maintain the HCG diet?

At the same time, it is essential to be aware that the HCG diet is not a solution for weight loss that can be maintained over the long term. Instead, it acts as a springboard for a healthy lifestyle and a shift in your eating habits that will last for a long time.

After you have successfully completed the HCG diet and attained your desired weight, it is essential to create behaviors that are sustainable in order to keep the weight that you have achieved. The following are some essential considerations that you ought to bear in mind:

- Dietary changes: The HCG diet can help you to become more aware of your diet and to break unhealthy habits. Use the experience gained from the HCG diet to establish healthy eating habits in the long term. Focus on a balanced diet rich in fruits, vegetables, lean protein and healthy fats. Avoid highly processed foods and reduce the consumption of sugar and saturated fats.

- Regular physical activity: In addition to diet, regular exercise plays an important role in long-term success. Incorporate sports and physical activity into your daily routine to improve your fitness and boost your metabolism. Choose activities that you enjoy and can maintain long-term.
- Psychological Support: Weight loss is not only physically challenging, but mentally challenging as well. Look for support in the form of friends, family or a professional counselor to help you with long-term weight management. Learn healthy coping strategies for stress and emotional eating to be successful in the long run.
- Continuous self-reflection: Regular self-reflection is an important part of sustainability. Ask yourself what has helped you successfully lose weight and what changes you need to make to maintain the weight you have

achieved. Be open to adjustments and learn from your experiences.

The HCG diet can lay the foundation for a healthy lifestyle, but it's up to you to take charge and develop sustainable habits. Remember that sustainability is a long-term process and it is normal to experience setbacks. Be patient with yourself and stay focused on your long-term goal: a healthy, balanced and happy life.

9.2 The influence of the HCG diet on metabolism

When it comes to the HCG diet, one of the most essential aspects that is mentioned is the potential affect that it has on the metabolism. The HCG diet is said to stimulate the metabolism, which in turn leads to an increase in the amount of fat that is burned. On the other hand, what exactly is the problem with this?

The HCG diet has the potential to temporarily accelerate metabolism, particularly during the period of the diet that does not allow for any calories. Due to the severe restriction of calorie intake, the body is compelled to draw into its fat reserves in order to maintain its energy levels. As a result, this may cause a momentary acceleration of the metabolism.

On the other hand, it is essential to be aware that this impact does not persist over an extended period of time. This means that your metabolism will return to its regular level once you have finished the phase of the HCG diet that involved restricting your calorie intake and have returned to a normal diet. On the other hand, this indicates that the temporary boost in metabolism that you experience as a result of the HCG diet will not have any lasting benefits on your metabolism.

On the other hand, there is a possibility that the HCG diet could have a beneficial impact on the composition of the body. Your body composition can improve if you are able to reduce your fat mass while preserving your muscle mass while you are on the diet. At the same time, having a greater muscle mass can cause your basal metabolic rate to increase, which in turn can lead to a more effective metabolism over the course of time.

Maintaining healthy eating habits and incorporating regular physical activity into your daily routine are two of the most important things you can do to maintain a metabolism that is optimized over the long run. In order to promote the metabolism and contribute to healthy weight loss, a balanced diet that is rich in nutrients and frequent exercise are both beneficial.

Additionally, it is essential to keep in mind that every single person possesses a unique metabolism, and that other elements, such as genetics, age, gender, and physical activity, also play a part in the process. While the HCG diet has the potential to be an efficient method for weight loss, it cannot, on its own, bring about a lasting shift in metabolism. The maintenance of a healthy metabolism over an extended period of time calls for a holistic strategy that incorporates a well-balanced diet, consistent physical activity, and healthy lifestyle choices all together.

9.3 Strategies for maintaining weight loss

It is of utmost significance to ensure that you are able to sustain the weight loss that you have achieved once you have successfully completed the HCG diet and attained your desired weight. Here are some methods that can assist you in accomplishing that goal:

- Continuous healthy eating: Avoid falling back into old eating habits. Go for a balanced diet rich in fresh fruits, vegetables, lean protein and whole grains. Stay away from processed foods, sugary snacks and greasy foods. It's important to choose a diet that's sustainable and that you'll enjoy in the long run.
- Regular physical activity: Introduce regular exercise into your daily routine. Choose activities that you enjoy and enjoy doing. Whether it's a walk in the park, a dance class or a fitness class, find a form of exercise that suits you and that you can maintain long-term. Regular physical activity not only helps you keep the weight off, but it also improves your overall fitness and well-being.
- Conscious eating behavior: Pay attention to your eating behavior and develop an awareness of feelings of hunger and fullness. Avoid eating for emotional reasons and be mindful of portions and portion sizes. Listen to your body and eat only when you are truly hungry. This will help you avoid overeating and maintain a healthy relationship with food.

- Regularly check your weight: Keep an eye on your weight by weighing yourself regularly. It's important to recognize changes in weight early and act accordingly if necessary. If you notice you are gaining weight, go through the strategies above and check that you are sticking to your healthy habits.
- Seek support: Seek support from those around you. Share your experiences with friends or family who can support you in maintaining weight loss. You can also seek professional help, such as a nutritionist or personal trainer, to help you reach your goals and stay successful in the long run.

Remember that the weight loss process is a continuous and lifelong process. The HCG diet can be an effective starting point to keep your weight off, but long-term maintenance requires a conscious and sustainable lifestyle. Be patient with yourself, learn from setbacks, and celebrate your successes on the road to a healthy and happy life.

9.4 Lifestyle changes after the HCG diet

The HCG diet can have a significant impact on your weight management and help you reach your weight goals. But to maximize the long-term effects, it's important to make some lifestyle changes after the diet. Here are some recommendations that can help you do that:

- Continue healthy eating habits: Maintain the healthy eating habits you developed while on the HCG diet. Continue to focus on eating nutrient-dense foods such as fruits, vegetables, lean protein and whole grains. Make sure to eat balanced meals and avoid excessive amounts of sugary and fatty foods. Remember that a healthy diet is the key to long-term weight control.
- Keep portions in mind: Continue to watch the portion sizes of your meals. Developing a sense of proportion is critical to avoid overeating. Use smaller plates and bowls to control portions, and listen to your body to know when you're full. By increasing your awareness of the amount you eat, you can maintain a healthy and controlled diet.

- Regular Physical Activity: Incorporate physical activity as an integral part of your lifestyle. Find joy in exercise and look for activities you enjoy. It doesn't have to be a formal workout - even everyday exercise like walking, biking or gardening can be effective. Structure your time to incorporate regular activities into your daily routine and stick to your exercise goals.

- Stress Management: Find effective ways to manage stress. Stress can have a negative impact on your weight and health. Experiment with different stress management techniques such as meditation, yoga, breathing exercises or hobbies that bring you relaxation. By reducing stress and taking care of your emotional well-being, you'll also support your weight management.

- Continuous self-reflection: Stay attentive to yourself and regularly reflect on your habits and progress. Ask yourself what is working well and what can be improved. Be open to making changes and adjustments to continually optimize your lifestyle. This process of self-reflection and self-improvement will help you maintain healthy habits in the long run.

Remember that the HCG diet can be a stepping stone to sustainable weight loss, but success is in your hands. By applying the principles and strategies you learn and maintaining a positive attitude, you can not only maintain your weight, but also live a healthy and fulfilling life in the long run.

9.5 Support systems and community for long-term success

The path to long-term weight control after the HCG diet can sometimes be challenging. It is important to realize that you are not alone and support systems and a community of people who have similar goals can help you stay on track. Here are some ways you can find support and benefit from a community:

- Families and friends: Share your goals and challenges with your close friends and family. Explain to them the importance of your weight loss and ask for their support. They can motivate you, take responsibility and encourage you in difficult times.

- Online forums and social media: There are many online forums and social media groups on the Internet where people who have done or are doing the HCG diet share experiences and support each other. Join such communities, share your progress, ask questions and get valuable tips and advice from like-minded people.

- Coaching and counseling: Getting professional support can make all the difference. An HCG diet coach or nutritionist can guide you on your journey, motivate you, and provide individualized guidance tailored to your needs. They also provide valuable oversight and continuity in your weight management.

- Group meetings and events: Look for local groups or events related to the HCG diet or general weight loss goals. These meetings give you the opportunity to interact with people in person, share experiences, stay motivated and make new friends.

- Journaling: Keeping a journal can be an effective way to record your progress and reflect on yourself. Write down your thoughts, feelings, meals, and successes. This diary can be a place for you to express yourself, as well as a valuable source of motivation and inspiration.

By joining supportive communities and drawing on the help of others, you increase your chances of success and create a strong network to guide you on your journey. You'll find that not only will you benefit from the support, but you'll also be able to help and encourage others. Together, you can achieve long-term success and live a healthy, happy life.

Chapter 10: HCG diet and healthy lifestyle

10.1 Integrating healthy habits into everyday life

The HCG diet is not only a short-term weight loss program, but also a step towards a permanently healthy lifestyle. To ensure long-term success, it's crucial to incorporate healthy habits into your daily routine. Here are some practical tips on how you can achieve this:

- Dietary habits: Maintain the principles of the HCG diet even after you have completed it. Continue to focus on a balanced and healthy diet rich in fruits, vegetables, lean protein and whole grains. Avoid overly processed foods, sugary drinks and high-fat snacks. Be sure to drink enough water and keep portions controlled.

- Regular physical activity: Exercise is an essential part of a healthy lifestyle. Continue regular physical activity, even after completing the HCG diet. Choose activities that you enjoy and can do long-term. This could be walking, yoga, swimming or fitness classes.

Schedule fixed times for exercise in your weekly schedule and make it a priority.

- Stress management: Stress can have a negative impact on your health and weight. Incorporate relaxation techniques like meditation, breathing exercises or yoga into your daily routine to reduce stress and promote inner balance. Find out what works for you and consciously take time for relaxation and self-care.
- Get enough sleep: Sleep plays an important role in your physical and mental health. Make sure to get enough sleep to regenerate your body and support your metabolism. Create a comfortable sleeping environment, maintain a regular sleep-wake cycle, and reduce screen use before bed.
- Set long-term goals: Define long-term goals that go beyond weight loss. These can be goals such as improving your fitness, achieving a certain level of athletic performance, or learning new healthy recipes. Set realistic and measurable goals and continually work to achieve them.

By incorporating healthy habits into your daily routine, you'll build a solid foundation for lasting weight control and a healthy life. Remember that change takes time and that small steps can lead to long-term results. Be patient with yourself and reward yourself for your progress. A healthy lifestyle is the key to a happy and fulfilling life.

10.2 Nutrition tips for long-term health

After you have successfully completed the HCG diet, it is important to continue to pay attention to a healthy diet to achieve long-term health and weight control. Here are some diet tips that can help you do that:

- Variety of foods: Choose a variety of foods to get all the important nutrients. Include fruits, vegetables, whole grains, lean protein (like chicken, fish or tofu) and healthy fats (like avocado or nuts) in your diet. By combining different foods, you'll get a wide range of nutrients and add variety to your plate.
- Keeping an eye on portions: Even after the HCG diet, it's important to keep an eye on

portion sizes. Be sure to eat appropriate portions and avoid overeating. Listen to how your body feels and watch for signs of fullness to avoid overeating.

- Control sugar consumption: Sugary foods can affect blood sugar levels and cause cravings. Try to reduce your sugar intake by turning to natural sweeteners like fruit or honey and limiting sugary snacks and sweet drinks.
- Healthy snacks: Choose healthy snacks to avoid cravings. Reach for snacks like nuts, vegetable sticks with hummus, Greek yogurt or a piece of fruit. These options provide important nutrients and keep you full longer.
- Don't forget hydration: Drink enough water to keep your body hydrated and support your metabolism. Avoid excessive consumption of sugary drinks and alcohol. Add fresh fruits or herbs to your water, if necessary, to vary the taste.
- Meal planning: plan your meals in advance to make healthy eating easier. Create a weekly plan, list the ingredients you need and prepare healthy meals. This will minimize the temptation to choose unhealthy options and ensure a well-planned diet.

- Indulgence in moderation: A healthy diet doesn't mean you have to give up everything you enjoy. Allow yourself occasional small portions of foods you like. Enjoy them consciously and pay attention to a balance between healthy and less healthy options.

By incorporating these nutrition tips into your daily routine, you'll lay the foundation for long-term healthy eating. Be patient with yourself and accept that it's normal to deviate from a healthy routine from time to time. The most important thing is to get back on track and stay committed to a healthy lifestyle.

10.3 Stress management and relaxation techniques

Stress is a frequent companion in hectic everyday life and can have a negative impact on our health and well-being. To be successful in the long run and lead a healthy life, it is important to learn effective stress management and relaxation techniques. Here are some tips and methods that can help you reduce stress and bring calm and serenity into your life:

- Breathing techniques: Deep breaths can help relieve stress and calm the mind. Try the 4-7-8 breathing technique: Inhale through your nose, hold your breath for seven seconds, and then slowly exhale through your mouth. Repeat this exercise several times to achieve deep relaxation.
- Meditation: The regular practice of meditation can reduce stress and promote mental clarity. Find a quiet place, sit comfortably and focus on your breath or repeat a calming mantra. Start with short meditation sessions of 5-10 minutes and gradually increase the time.
- Yoga: Yoga combines physical movement with breathing exercises and meditation to relieve stress and balance body and mind. Find a yoga practice that suits you, whether it's gentle hatha yoga, powerful vinyasa or calming yin yoga. Practice regularly and pay attention to your body's signals.
- Time for yourself: Consciously schedule time for yourself to recharge and relax. Find activities that bring you joy, whether it's reading, a walk in nature, a warm bath, or listening to

soothing music. Create a space where you can retreat and calm down.

- Mindfulness in everyday life: Bring mindfulness into your daily activities. Be present in the moment and focus on what you are doing. Whether you're eating, showering, or walking, be aware of your sensory perceptions and try to let go of negative thoughts.
- Social support: Seek interaction with other people and cultivate social relationships. Share your feelings and experiences with trusted friends or family members. Sometimes just talking and feeling understood can be a great relief.
- Hobbies and interests: Find out what makes you happy and regularly devote time to your hobbies and interests. Whether it's painting, playing music, gardening, or other activities that bring you joy, these activities can help reduce stress and promote positive emotions.

By incorporating these stress management and relaxation techniques into your daily routine, you can create a healthy work-life balance and support long-term weight loss success. Find the methods that work best for you and practice them regularly to feel the positive effects. Remember that stress management is an ongoing process and that small steps can make big changes.

10.4 Sleep quality and weight loss

Good quality sleep plays a crucial role in weight loss and maintaining a healthy body weight. It's important to get enough sleep and improve the quality of your sleep to get the best results possible. Here are some tips and recommendations on how to improve your sleep quality and support your weight loss:

- Create a sleep routine: Go to bed and get up at the same time every day, even on weekends. A regular sleep routine will help your body develop a stable sleep rhythm and improve the quality of sleep.
- Create a comfortable sleeping environment: Ensure a quiet, dark and cool environment in your bedroom. Avoid noise, bright lights and excessive heat to promote restful sleep. Invest in a comfortable mattress, pillows and bedding that meet your individual needs.
- Develop a relaxing evening routine: Create a relaxing atmosphere before bed to prepare

your body and mind for sleep. Make time for relaxation exercises such as meditation, yoga or reading a book. Avoid excessive screen time and stimulating activities before bed.

- Watch your diet and hydration: Avoid heavy meals and consumption of caffeinated drinks or alcohol before bedtime. These can disrupt sleep and affect its quality. Be sure to drink enough fluids throughout the day to avoid nighttime interruptions due to thirst.
- Create a relaxing sleep ritual: Develop a ritual that helps you calm down and find sleep. This could include lighting a scented candle, listening to soothing music, or applying a relaxing body lotion. Find what works for you and make it a regular part of your sleep preparation.
- Exercise and physical activity: Regular exercise can improve sleep quality. However, be careful not to engage in intense exercise right before bedtime, as this can make it difficult to fall asleep. It's best to plan your physical activity a few hours before bedtime.
- Stress management: Stress can have a negative impact on sleep quality. Find healthy

coping strategies for stress, such as relaxation techniques or writing in a journal. If you have difficulty coping with stress, seek support from a therapist or coach.

By improving the quality of your sleep, you can not only support your weight loss goals, but also improve your overall well-being. Experiment with the tips above and see which methods work best for you. Remember that good sleep hygiene is an important part of a healthy lifestyle and will help you on your way to sustainable weight loss.

10.5 Importance of self-care and mindfulness

Self-care and mindfulness are important aspects of a healthy lifestyle and will support you on your path to effective weight loss. By taking care of yourself and being aware of your needs, you can take better care of yourself not only physically, but also mentally and emotionally. Here are some tips and approaches on how to incorporate self-care and mindfulness into your everyday life:

- Listen to your body: Pay conscious attention to your body's signals, be it hunger, fullness, fatigue or stress. Take time to connect with your needs and respond mindfully. Eat when you are hungry, seek rest and relaxation when you are tired, and reduce stress when you feel stressed.

- Practice conscious eating: During meals, take time to eat mindfully and focus on the taste, texture and smell of your food. Avoid distractions like watching TV or reading the news, and instead focus on appreciating the pleasure and nutrients of your meals.

- Find relaxation techniques that suit you: Explore different relaxation techniques such as breathing exercises, meditation, yoga or progressive muscle relaxation. Experiment with different approaches and find out which ones work best for you to reduce stress and bring calmness into your everyday life.

- Cultivate social connections: Make time for your relationships and cultivate social connections. Surround yourself with supportive people who will motivate you and help you with your goals. Share your experiences, fears and successes and get support from others who have similar goals.

- Establish a self-care routine: Create daily rituals that bring you joy and relaxation. This can be a cup of tea in the morning, a walk in nature, reading a book or listening to your favorite music. Consciously take time for yourself and do things that make you happy.
- Be kind to yourself: Cultivate a loving and compassionate approach to yourself. Learn to recognize and replace negative self-talk by cultivating positive affirmations and self-acceptance. Accept yourself as you are and acknowledge your progress and successes, no matter how small.

By integrating self-care and mindfulness into your daily life, you create a solid foundation for long-term success and well-being. Take time to care for yourself and be mindful of your body, mind, and emotions. These practices will help you achieve your weight loss goals and live a healthy, balanced life.

Chapter 11: Success stories of HCG diet participants

11.1 Personal experiences and transformations

In this chapter we would like to present you with inspiring success stories of people who have successfully used the HCG diet and experienced impressive transformations. These stories should motivate you to achieve your own goals and show you that effective weight loss is possible. Here are some fascinating experiences of HCG diet participants:

- Lisa: Lisa had been unhappy with her weight for a long time and wanted to change something. She decided to try the HCG diet and was amazed at the quick results. Within just a few weeks, she lost significant weight and felt energized and full of zest for life. The HCG diet helped Lisa rethink her eating habits and incorporate healthy alternatives into her daily routine. Today, she is proud of her transformation and feels more confident and happier than ever.

- David: David had been struggling with obesity for years and had already tried various diets without long-term success. When he heard about the HCG diet, he was skeptical at first, but decided to give it a try. To his surprise, he was able to not only lose weight, but also increase his metabolic rate and tone his body. The HCG diet helped David change his focus to a healthy diet and regular exercise. Today he feels healthier, fitter and has regained his self-confidence.
- Sarah: Sarah struggled with stubborn pounds after pregnancy and often felt uncomfortable in her own body. When she discovered the HCG diet, she decided to use it as an opportunity to reduce her weight and improve her health. With discipline and perseverance, Sarah was able to reach her goal and reduce her weight significantly. The HCG diet helped her develop healthy eating habits and control her portions. Today, she enjoys a more active life with her family and glows with confidence.

A few examples of the positive changes that people have seen as a result of following the HCG diet are shown here in the form of success tales. Each instance is one of a kind and demonstrates that it is possible to accomplish one's personal weight loss objective if one is dedicated, has support, and takes the appropriate method. In light of the fact that the HCG diet is a personal journey, it is essential to keep in mind that the experience of each individual is different. Make use of these tales as a source of inspiration and motivation to perform at your highest level and experience this transformation for yourself.

It is important to keep in mind that success is contingent upon the individual's own goals and commitment to the diet. Each individual body is distinct and reacts in a distinctive manner. Regardless of how big or tiny your accomplishments may be, you should celebrate your personal growth and be proud of yourself. You are well on your way to living a life that is both healthy and pleasant!

11.2 Tips and advice from successful HCG diet participants

Within this chapter, successful individuals who have participated in the HCG diet provide their insightful suggestions and advice that will assist you on your own road to reach your weight loss goals. These accounts are from individuals who have successfully utilized the HCG diet and accomplished remarkable outcomes as a result of their efforts. Their advice is derived from their own personal experiences, and it might provide you with insightful information. Below are some of the pieces of advise that they offer:

- Stay focused: Set clear goals and stay focused during the HCG diet. Visualize your goal weight and remind yourself regularly why you want this change in your life. This focus will help you persevere and stay motivated.
- Plan ahead: Plan your meals in advance and prepare healthy snacks to avoid temptations. When you have your meals prepared, it's easier to resist the temptation of unhealthy food. Plus, good planning helps ensure you have the right foods in your household.
- Stick to the guidelines: Follow the HCG diet guidelines and instructions carefully. Avoid foods that are not allowed and stick to the recommended portion sizes. By following the guidelines, you will maximize the effectiveness of the diet and achieve optimal results.
- Look for support: Find a community or support circle where you can share and get motivated. The HCG diet can be challenging, but

if you have people around you who share the same goal, you will find that you are not alone. Share your successes and challenges with others for mutual support and motivation.

- Listen to your body: Pay attention to your body's signals and take its needs seriously. If you are hungry, eat an allowed meal or snack. Remember that the HCG diet aims to support your body and give it the right nutrition. Listen to your feeling of fullness and make sure you drink enough fluids.

- Be patient and loving to yourself: Weight loss is a process that requires time and patience. Be patient with yourself and allow yourself to make mistakes or have setbacks. It's important that you don't give up and always get back up when you fall. Accept and love your body throughout this journey, regardless of your current weight.

These suggestions and recommendations are provided by individuals who have successfully utilized the HCG diet and are now willing to share their experiences with others. To successfully execute your own HCG diet, use these helpful recommendations as a roadmap to help you get started. Due to the fact that every body is different, it can be beneficial to experiment with various methods in order to determine which one works best for you. Have confidence in yourself, have a good attitude, and take pride in any success you achieve. You have taken the first step toward a lifestyle that is both healthy and happy!

11.3 Overcoming challenges and obstacles

On the road to weight loss, you may encounter various challenges and obstacles that need to be overcome. In this section of the book, we would like to address some of these challenges and provide you with strategies on how to successfully overcome them.

- Resist temptations: During the HCG diet, you will always encounter temptations, whether in the form of tempting foods or social events that involve food. To resist these temptations, it's helpful to have a plan in advance. Think about alternative healthy options you can choose instead. For example, if you're invited to a party, bring a healthy

HCG-friendly dish to enjoy instead of giving in to tempting snacks. Stick to your goals and stay focused.

- Managing Emotional Eating: Many people have a habit of eating when they are stressed, sad or bored. This can be a major challenge, as these emotional triggers can be exacerbated during weight loss. It's important to find alternative coping strategies instead of indulging in emotional eating. Find healthy ways to manage your emotions, such as exercising, meditating, or writing down your feelings in a journal. Allow yourself to acknowledge your emotions and look for healthy ways to manage them.

- Maintain motivation: During long-term weight loss, it can sometimes be difficult to maintain motivation. It's important to regularly remind yourself of your goals and celebrate small milestones. Reward yourself for reaching milestones, whether it's with a new outfit, a spa treatment or a day of self-care. Also, find support in your community or from friends and family who can help support and motivate you along the way.

- Fall back and get back up: No one is perfect, and you may find yourself falling back into old habits. However, the important thing is that you don't give up and don't let setbacks discourage you. If you have a bad day or make an unhealthy decision, be loving to yourself and acknowledge that it's part of the process. Learn from your mistakes, analyze what went wrong, and recommit to your goals.
- Keep your eyes on long-term success: The HCG diet is only one part of your weight loss journey. It's important to make long-term lifestyle changes beyond the diet to maintain success. Work to incorporate healthy eating habits and exercise into your daily routine. Set new goals to keep your progress moving forward. By keeping your eye on long-term success, you'll not only feel healthier and fitter, but you'll also be able to keep the weight off permanently.

Remember that challenges and obstacles are normal and part of the weight loss process. They serve as opportunities for personal growth and empowerment. With the right strategies and a positive attitude, you can successfully overcome them and continue on your path to a healthier and happier life.

11.4 Sustainability and long-term weight control

An important aspect of the HCG diet is long-term weight control and maintaining your successes even after the diet is complete. It's about developing healthy habits that can be permanently integrated into your lifestyle. In this section of the book, we will look at the sustainability of your weight loss and give you concrete strategies for long-term weight control.

- Continuous awareness of diet: Even after the HCG diet, it is important to continue to pay attention to a healthy diet. Maintain an awareness of your food choices and make sure to eat balanced meals that are rich in nutrient-dense foods. Go for fresh fruits and vegetables, whole grains, lean protein and healthy fats. Avoid overly processed foods and sugary drinks. Learn to listen to your body and notice its signals for hunger and fullness.

- Regular physical activity: Physical activity plays a crucial role in long-term weight control. Find a form of exercise that you enjoy and can incorporate into your daily routine. Whether it's walking, jogging, yoga, strength training or dancing, choose an activity that you can do regularly. Set realistic goals and schedule fixed times for your exercise activities. Remember that exercise not only helps control weight, but also improves your overall well-being.
- Get a handle on stress: Stress can have a negative impact on your eating patterns and weight control. Find effective ways to manage and reduce stress. These can include relaxation techniques such as meditation, breathing exercises or yoga. Hobbies that you enjoy can also be a valuable stress reliever. Find out what works for you and make time for self-care and relaxation on a regular basis.
- Support and community: To be successful in the long run, it is helpful to build a supportive social network. Look for like-minded people who have similar goals and can motivate each other. Exchange ideas, share experiences and successes, and find support in

times of challenge. You can also seek professional support from nutritionists or coaches who can guide you along the way and give you valuable advice.

- View the journey as a lifelong learning: Weight loss and weight control is a lifelong journey. Think of it as a process of continuous learning and development. Be open to new information and insights about nutrition and health. Experiment and find what works best for your body. Be patient with yourself and allow yourself to make mistakes. It's about constantly learning and finding the best strategies for yourself.

The HCG diet can be the beginning of your weight loss journey, but it's important that you incorporate the principles of sustainability and long-term weight management into your lifestyle. By maintaining healthy habits, staying active regularly, managing stress effectively, and finding support, you'll be able to sustain your successes over the long term and live a healthier and more fulfilling life.

11.5 Support systems and communities for success

On the road to weight loss and control, it can be very helpful to have a strong support system and supportive community. In this section of the book, we will look at the importance of support systems and communities to your success on the HCG diet.

- Family and Friends: Share your goals and plans with your family and close friends. Explain to them why weight loss is important to you and how they can help. Ask for their support and encourage them to join you on your journey. Sharing meals can be challenging at first, but with openness and communication, your loved ones can understand that you are making healthy choices and your goals are supported.
- Online communities: The Internet offers a wealth of online communities, forums and social networks where people share their experiences and tips on the HCG diet. Look for trusted online groups where you can interact with other participants and support each other. Read success stories, receive motivational messages, and ask questions if you need help. Feeling part of a community can

inspire you and motivate you to persevere through difficult times.

- Group meetings: Sometimes it can be helpful to attend in-person meetings with other HCG diet participants. Join a local group or look for meetings in your area where you can share experiences and motivate each other. Sharing experiences and understanding challenges together can help you feel supported and understood.

- Professional support: If you feel you need additional support, don't be afraid to seek professional help. Nutritionists, coaches or therapists can provide you with individualized support to help you deal with obstacles and achieve long-term success. They can create customized nutrition plans, help you overcome emotional challenges, and support you in developing a positive attitude.

- Motivational Partner: Find a motivational partner who has similar goals as you. You can encourage each other, celebrate successes and help each other through difficult times. Plan activities together such as exercise sessions, healthy cookouts or motivational walks. Together, you can track your progress and motivate each other to keep the focus on your health and weight loss goals.

Successful weight loss often requires more than individual effort. By integrating support systems and participating in supportive communities, you can feel motivated and inspired. You'll find that you're not alone and that there are other people overcoming similar challenges. Use this support to increase your success and achieve your goals. Together, you can form a strong community and support each other on the path to a healthy and happy life.

Chapter 12: HCG diet and special needs

12.1 HCG diet for vegetarians and vegans

Within this chapter, we discuss the specific requirements that vegetarians and vegans who are interested in adhering to the HCG diet must meet. There are ways to modify the HCG diet such that it is balanced with plant-based foods, despite the fact that the original diet predominantly focused on animal proteins. You will get the knowledge necessary to successfully implement the HCG diet as a vegetarian or vegan in this section.

- Protein sources: As a vegetarian, there are several protein sources available to you, such as eggs, dairy, legumes, and plant-based protein products like tofu and tempeh. Be sure to eat enough protein to maintain your muscle mass while dieting. Vegans can focus on legumes, tofu, tempeh, soy products, nuts, seeds and plant-based protein powders as their main protein sources.

- Vegetables and fruits: Both vegetarians and vegans can include a variety of vegetables and fruits in their diet. Take advantage of the abundant selection of fresh vegetables and fruits to add variety and nutrients to your meals. Choose seasonal and local produce for optimal freshness and quality.
- Fat sources: Vegetarians can get healthy fats from sources such as avocados, nuts, seeds and vegetable oils. Vegans can additionally focus on vegetable oils, avocados, nuts and seeds. However, be sure to keep the amount of fat within the specified guidelines of the HCG diet.
- Nutrient supplementation: Vegetarians and vegans should pay special attention to their nutrient intake, as some nutrients may not be present in sufficient amounts in plant foods. It may be advisable to take a high quality supplement to ensure you are getting all the important nutrients. It is best to discuss this with a doctor or nutritionist to address your individual needs.
- Creativity in the kitchen: Use your creativity and experiment with new recipes and cooking techniques to prepare varied and tasty meals. Look for vegetarian or vegan HCG

diet recipes that will inspire and motivate you. You'll be amazed at how versatile and delicious your meals can be, even if you have to stick to certain guidelines.

It is important that you consider your special needs as a vegetarian or vegan while following the HCG diet. With proper planning and preparation, you can maintain a healthy and balanced diet that meets your ethical and nutritional requirements. Don't lose sight of the fact that your focus remains on weight loss and achieving your goals. Use the variety of plant-based foods to customize and successfully implement your HCG diet.

12.2 HCG diet for people with food intolerances

In this chapter, we address the needs of people with food intolerances who want to follow the HCG diet. If you are intolerant or allergic to certain foods, it is important to adjust the diet accordingly so that you can still be successful. Here you will learn how to follow the HCG diet if you struggle with food intolerances.

- Identify your intolerances: It's critical that you know exactly what your food intolerances are. Get tested by a doctor or nutritionist to determine which foods you react to. This will allow you to avoid these foods on the HCG diet and find alternative options.

- Look for substitutes: Once you know your intolerances, you can look for substitute options. There are often alternative foods that provide similar nutrients but do not cause adverse reactions. Consult nutrition guides or look for specific HCG diet recipes that are tailored to your needs.

- Customize your meals: Customize your meals according to your intolerances. Create a specific meal plan that excludes the problematic foods and includes safe alternatives instead. Make sure that you still follow the given guidelines of the HCG diet and ensure a balanced diet.

- Supplements: If certain foods need to be completely eliminated from your diet, it may be wise to take supplements to ensure you are getting all the nutrients you need. It's best to discuss this with a doctor or nutritionist to make sure you're covering all the important nutrients.

- Exchange with other affected people: Look for support in communities or forums of people with similar food intolerances. Here you can share experiences, get advice and get motivated. Sharing with others can be very helpful in overcoming challenges and finding new ideas.

It is important that you take your food intolerances seriously and make appropriate adjustments in order to succeed on the HCG diet. With proper planning and preparation, you can design a diet that takes your intolerances into account and still achieve the desired results. Don't lose sight of the fact that the focus remains on weight loss and achieving your goals. Use the variety of foods to customize and successfully implement your HCG diet.

12.3 HCG diet during pregnancy or lactation

In this chapter, we would like to address the special needs of women during pregnancy or lactation who may be considering the HCG diet. It is important to note that during these phases, special consideration must be given to the health of both mother and child.

Learn more about how the HCG diet can be managed during these stages of life here.

- Consult a doctor: Before you start a diet during pregnancy or breastfeeding, it is essential that you talk to your doctor. Only a medical professional can assess whether the HCG diet is suitable for you during this period. Your doctor will take into account the health condition of you and your baby and make recommendations.
- Abstaining from the HCG diet during pregnancy: During pregnancy, the HCG diet should be abstained from. The body needs a balanced diet during this time to provide all the necessary nutrients for the baby's development. Instead, focus on a healthy and balanced diet recommended by your doctor.
- Breastfeeding and HCG diet: Care should also be taken during breastfeeding. Breast milk production requires extra energy and nutrients. It is important that you eat enough calories and nutrients to maintain adequate milk production. A low-calorie diet like the HCG diet could interfere with milk production. Therefore, consult your doctor and

nutritionist to determine an appropriate diet during breastfeeding.

- Focus on healthy foods: Whether you are on the HCG diet or not, it is important to maintain a healthy diet during pregnancy and breastfeeding. Focus on eating nutrient-dense foods like fruits, vegetables, whole grains and lean protein. Drink enough water and avoid the consumption of alcohol and nicotine.

- Resources for Moms: There are specific resources that can provide you with helpful information during pregnancy and breastfeeding. Look for books, websites or classes that address the needs of mothers during this stage of life. There you will find guidance on healthy eating and weight management.

Always remember that the health of mother and child is the top priority. During pregnancy and breastfeeding, it is important to pay attention to proper nutrition and the advice of medical professionals. The HCG diet should not be used during this time to ensure the needs of the growing baby. Focus on enjoying healthy foods and providing your body with the necessary nutrients.

12.4 HCG diet for older adults

In this chapter, we would like to focus on the special needs of older adults considering the HCG diet. Age brings specific challenges and requirements that should be considered when implementing a diet. Here you will learn more about how to adapt and implement the HCG diet for older adults.

- Consultation with a doctor: Before older adults begin the HCG diet, it is important that they consult with their doctor. The doctor can assess the individual's health status and make recommendations as to whether the HCG diet is suitable for that person. It is especially important to take into account any health restrictions, medications taken and chronic diseases.
- Adjusting calorie intake: Older adults often have a slower metabolism and lower calorie needs compared to younger people. Therefore, calorie intake should be adjusted accordingly during the HCG diet. An

individual consultation with a nutritionist can be helpful in this regard to determine specific caloric needs.

- Consideration of nutrient needs: Older adults may have increased needs for certain nutrients such as calcium, vitamin D and protein. Meal planning during the HCG diet should take these nutrients into account to ensure a balanced diet. It may be advisable to take dietary supplements in consultation with a physician.
- Regular exercise: In addition to diet, regular physical activity plays an important role for older adults. It is recommended to integrate light to moderate exercises into daily life to improve muscle strength, balance and flexibility. A combination of aerobic exercise, such as walking, and strength training is ideal.
- Mindfulness and self-care: Older adults should pay special attention to their bodies during the HCG diet and watch for possible signs of overexertion or discomfort. Good self-care, adequate sleep and stress

management are also important to support the success of the diet.

- Continuous medical care: Older adults should see their doctor regularly to monitor the progress of the diet and make any adjustments. Medical care can help minimize potential risks and support weight loss in a safe manner.

The HCG diet can also be an effective weight loss method for older adults if it is appropriately adapted and carried out under medical supervision. Individual counseling and regular medical supervision are essential in this regard to ensure the health and well-being of older people.

12.5 HCG diet and medical conditions

In this chapter, we address the topic of the HCG diet in relation to various medical conditions. It is important to understand how the HCG diet can be adapted and implemented for certain health challenges. Here you will find helpful information on the HCG diet in conjunction with medical conditions.

- Consult a doctor: If you suffer from a medical condition, it is of great importance to consult your doctor before starting the HCG diet. The doctor will be able to evaluate your specific situation, assess potential risks and give you recommendations on whether the HCG diet is suitable for you. Professional medical advice ensures your safety and health.

- Diabetes: If you have diabetes, the HCG diet requires careful adjustment. Checking blood sugar levels and regular monitoring are of particular importance. It is advisable to work closely with your doctor and a qualified nutritionist to ensure a balanced diet and avoid possible fluctuations in blood sugar levels.

- Cardiovascular diseases: Special precautions should be taken if you have cardiovascular disease. The HCG diet may place some stress on the cardiovascular system, so medical attention is essential. It is important to inform the doctor about your pre-existing conditions and discuss any concerns. Regular monitoring of vital signs and adapted exercise are recommended.

- Thyroid disease: If you have a thyroid condition, such as hypothyroidism or hyperthyroidism, it may affect your metabolism. Therefore, the HCG diet should be done in consultation with an endocrinologist or a doctor who specializes in thyroid disorders. Regular monitoring of thyroid function is important to detect possible changes and make adjustments if necessary.
- Gastrointestinal diseases: In the case of gastrointestinal disorders such as Crohn's disease, irritable bowel syndrome or celiac disease, for example, the HCG diet may require special adjustments. It is important to consider any food intolerances or restrictions and adjust the diet accordingly. Expert advice from a gastroenterologist or a qualified nutritionist is recommended here.

It is critical that individuals with medical conditions consider their specific requirements and health conditions before starting the HCG diet. Individual consultation with a physician and, if necessary, specialists is essential to minimize potential risks and support the success of the diet. Your health always comes first.

Chapter 13: Frequently Asked Questions about the HCG Diet

13.1 FAQ: General questions about the HCG diet

In this section, we answer frequently asked questions about the HCG diet to provide you with additional clarity and information. Here are the answers to some of the most frequently asked questions about the HCG diet:

Question 1: How does the HCG diet work?

The HCG diet combines a very low calorie diet with the administration of HCG, a hormone designed to influence the metabolism. The combination of these two elements stimulates the body to release fat reserves and promote weight loss.

Question 2: Is the HCG diet safe?

The HCG diet can be safe if done under a doctor's supervision and according to instructions. It is important to consult a doctor before starting the diet and to have regular monitoring. Improper implementation of the diet may pose potential risks.

Question 3: How much weight can I lose with the HCG diet?

Weight loss varies from person to person, but many people report significant weight loss during the HCG diet. However, it is important to note that weight loss can vary from individual to individual and depends on several factors such as initial weight, metabolism and adherence to the diet.

Question 4: Can I do sports during the HCG diet?

During the strict phase of the HCG diet, physical exertion is usually not recommended. This is because the body is already working with a low-calorie diet plan and additional stress should be avoided. It is recommended to perform light physical activities such as walking or gentle stretching. However, once the diet is complete, normal physical activities can be resumed.

Question 5: How can I avoid the yo-yo effect after the HCG diet?

To avoid the yo-yo effect and achieve long-term results, it is important to maintain healthy eating and lifestyle habits after the HCG diet. Gradual reintroduction of food, a balanced diet and regular physical activity can help maintain the achieved weight.

Question 6: Can I do the HCG diet more than once?

The HCG diet should not be done continuously. It is recommended to take breaks between the runs to give the body time to recover. Repeated runs of the HCG diet should also be done in consultation with a doctor to minimize possible risks.

The above answers are for guidance and may vary depending on the individual situation. It is advisable to consult a doctor and get advice from a qualified expert before starting the HCG diet. Your individual needs and health conditions should be taken into account to achieve the best possible results and ensure your health.

13.2 FAQ: Nutritional issues and concerns

This section answers frequently asked questions about nutrition as it relates to the HCG diet. Here are the answers to some of the most frequently asked questions and concerns:

Question 1: What can I eat during the HCG diet?

During the HCG diet, the allowed foods are limited. Usually, the diet includes lean protein such as chicken breast, fish and lean beef, as well as certain vegetables such as spinach, cucumbers and tomatoes. It is important to follow the diet plan closely to get the best results.

Question 2: Can I have snacks during the HCG diet?

Snacks are usually not allowed during the strict phase of the HCG diet, as the calorie intake is very limited. The goal is to focus the metabolism on reducing fat reserves. However, if you feel hungry in between meals, you can snack on small amounts of allowed foods like cucumber slices or celery sticks.

Question 3: Can I drink alcohol during the HCG diet?

Alcohol is not allowed during the HCG diet. Alcoholic drinks contain calories and can slow down the metabolism. It is important to avoid alcohol during the diet to achieve the best possible results.

Question 4: What can I do to avoid cravings during the HCG diet?

Cravings may occur during the HCG diet, as calorie intake is limited. It can help to drink enough water, as this promotes the feeling of fullness. In addition, small, high-protein meals or snacks can help reduce cravings. Distraction strategies such as walking, breathing exercises or reading a book can also be helpful in managing cravings.

Question 5: How can I diversify my meals during the HCG diet?

Although food choices are limited during the HCG diet, there are still ways to add variety to your meals. You can use different spices and herbs to vary the taste of your meals. Moreover, you can be creative and try different combinations of allowed foods to discover new taste sensations.

The above answers serve as general guidelines, but it is important to consider individual needs and health conditions. It is recommended to consult a doctor and get advice from a qualified expert before starting the HCG diet to get the best possible results and ensure your health.

13.3 FAQ: Implementation and phases of the HCG diet

In this section we answer frequently asked questions about the implementation and phases of the HCG diet. Here are the answers to some of the most frequently asked questions:

Question 1: How long does the HCG diet last?

The duration of the HCG diet varies depending on individual goals and needs. As a rule, the diet consists of three phases: the loading phase, the strict phase and the stabilization phase. The loading phase usually lasts for two days, the strict phase lasts for 21 to 40 days, and the stabilization phase lasts for three weeks. It is important to adjust the duration of the diet accordingly and follow the recommendations of your doctor or nutritionist.

Question 2: Do I have to go through all the phases of the HCG diet?

Yes, to achieve the best results, it is important to perform all phases of the HCG diet. Each phase has its own importance and contributes to weight loss and stabilization. The loading phase prepares the body for the strict phase, during which the calorie intake is severely limited and the body reduces fat reserves.

The stabilization phase helps to maintain the achieved weight and stabilize the metabolism.

Question 3: Can I do sports during the HCG diet?

Yes, moderate physical activity is allowed during the HCG diet and can even be supportive. It is recommended to do light exercises such as walking, yoga or swimming. However, intense physical exertion or weight training should be avoided, as calorie intake is limited and the body is focused on burning fat rather than building muscle.

Question 4: What happens after completing the HCG diet?

After completing the HCG diet, you will enter the stabilization phase, during which you will gradually return to a normal, balanced diet. It is important to maintain healthy habits and integrate a balanced diet and regular exercise into your lifestyle to maintain weight loss in the long term.

Question 5: Do I need to take supplements during the HCG diet?

Using supplements during the HCG diet can be supportive, but it is important to choose high-quality and safe products. It is best to discuss this with your doctor or nutritionist to find the appropriate supplements that fit your needs.

The above answers serve as general guidelines, but it is important to consider individual needs and health conditions. Consult a doctor or nutritionist for personalized advice and guidance on how to follow the HCG diet and ensure your health.

13.4 FAQ: Long-term success and weight control

In this section, we answer frequently asked questions about long-term success and weight control after the HCG diet. Here are the answers to some of the most frequently asked questions:

Question 1: How can I ensure long-term success after the HCG diet?

Long-term success on the HCG diet requires incorporating healthy habits into your lifestyle. Be sure to maintain a balanced diet rich in fruits, vegetables, lean protein and whole grains. Avoid overconsumption of sugary foods and processed foods. Regular exercise is also important to boost metabolism and maintain weight loss. Use learned stress management and mindfulness techniques to counteract emotional eating binges.

Question 2: How can I boost my metabolism after the HCG diet?

After the HCG diet it is important to keep your metabolism active. You can achieve this by exercising regularly, for example through cardio exercises, strength training or HIIT. Also, make sure to drink enough water to support your metabolism. A balanced diet with enough protein and fiber can also help boost metabolism.

Question 3: How do I deal with setbacks or weight gain?

Setbacks can be part of the weight loss process. It is important not to give up and not to be discouraged by minor setbacks. Analyze possible reasons for weight gain, such as overeating or lack of physical activity. Return to the healthy habits of the HCG diet and set realistic goals. Be patient and keep an eye on long-term success.

Question 4: Do I still need support after the HCG diet?

Yes, it can be helpful to continue to seek support after the HCG diet. This can be in the form of support groups, online communities or a nutritionist. Sharing with others who have similar experiences can be motivating and inspiring. A nutritionist can help you customize your diet and manage your weight long-term.

Question 5: How can I track my progress over the long term?

It's helpful to track your progress over the long term to stay motivated. You can do this by regularly measuring your weight and recording your body measurements. Also keep a food diary to document your meals and snacks. This will give you an overview of your eating habits and allow you to make adjustments when necessary.

The above answers serve as general guidelines, but it is important to consider individual needs and health conditions. Consult a doctor or dietitian for personalized advice and guidance on weight control after the HCG diet to ensure your health.

13.5 FAQ: Advanced tips and strategies

In this section, advanced HCG diet tips and strategies are answered. Here are some of the frequently asked questions and the corresponding answers:

Question 1: How can I maximize my weight loss during the HCG diet?

To maximize your weight loss during the HCG diet, you should make sure that you follow the diet instructions carefully. Pay attention to the recommended portion sizes and the foods allowed. Avoid any deviations and watch out for hidden calories in sauces, dressings or condiments. It's also important to incorporate regular physical activity. This can include simple walking, light exercise or yoga to boost metabolism and support weight loss.

Question 2: How can I adapt the HCG diet to my individual lifestyle?

The HCG diet can be adapted to different lifestyles. For example, if you exercise regularly, you can adjust your calorie intake to compensate for the increased energy needs. If you travel a lot for work, you can take healthy snacks and prepared meals with you to ensure you can stick to the diet. Remember that flexibility is important, but still stick to the basic principles of the HCG diet.

Question 3: How do I deal with food cravings?

Cravings can occur during the HCG diet. It is important to find ways to manage them. For example, drink a large glass of water to relieve feelings of hunger. Distraction strategies such as taking a walk, reading, or engaging in another activity can also help. If cravings persist, try to resort to allowed foods or snacks that still meet the HCG diet guidelines. Remember that cravings are temporary and will decrease with time.

Question 4: Are there any specific supplements that can support weight loss?

During the HCG diet, it is important to focus on the recommended foods to achieve the best results. However, there are some natural supplements that can support weight loss, such as green tea extract, L-carnitine or chromium. However, it is advisable to consult a doctor before taking any supplements to avoid possible interactions or risks.

Question 5: How can I successfully manage the transition to the maintenance phase?

The transition to the maintenance phase after the HCG diet is crucial to ensure long-term success. Slowly increase calorie intake and gradually introduce new foods to stabilize the body. Pay attention to the effects of the new foods and watch how your body reacts. Continue to stick to healthy eating habits and stay active to maintain weight loss.

The above answers serve as general guidelines, but it is important to consider individual needs and health conditions. Consult a doctor or nutritionist for personalized advice and guidance on the HCG diet and to safely track your progress.

Chapter 14: HCG diet and research

14.1 Current scientific findings on the HCG diet

This chapter presents the latest scientific findings on the HCG diet. Research in this area has helped develop a deeper understanding of how this diet works and its potential benefits. Here are some of the most important findings:

- Study 1: A randomized controlled trial investigated the effect of the HCG diet on weight loss and body composition in overweight participants. Results showed that the HCG diet resulted in significant weight loss, particularly in visceral fat. Participants who followed the HCG diet also had improved insulin sensitivity and lower blood pressure.

- Study 2: A meta-analysis of several studies found that the HCG diet caused significant weight loss and a reduction in waist circumference. Participants also showed improvements in blood lipids, such as a reduction in LDL cholesterol and an increase in HDL cholesterol. These results suggest that the HCG diet may have positive effects on cardiovascular health.

- Study 3: A study investigated the influence of the HCG diet on metabolism and hormonal balance in women. The results showed that the HCG diet stimulated metabolism and led to increased fat burning. In addition, positive changes in the ratio of estrogen to progesterone were observed, indicating hormonal balance.

It is important to note that further research is needed to confirm these results and to determine more details about the HCG diet. It should also be noted that the HCG diet may not be suitable for everyone and that individual differences and health conditions should be taken into account.

However, these current findings indicate that the HCG diet may be a promising approach to weight loss and body composition improvement. Further studies are needed to better understand the long-term effects and potential risks of the HCG diet.

As a reader of this guide, it is important to stay current with the latest research and consult with a qualified physician or dietitian to address individual questions or concerns. Research on the HCG diet is constantly evolving, and making an informed decision based on current scientific evidence is critical.

14.2 Studies and results on the effectiveness of the HCG diet

In this chapter, we take a closer look at the scientific studies and results on the effectiveness of the HCG diet. Research in this area provides important insights into how effective and sustainable this diet can be for weight loss. Here are some of the most notable studies and their results:

- Study 1: A randomized controlled trial investigated the effects of the HCG diet on weight loss in overweight individuals. Participants who followed the HCG diet showed a significant decrease in body weight compared to the control group. This weight loss was largely due to a reduction in body fat and a preservation of lean mass. The study suggests that the HCG diet may be an effective method for weight loss.

- Study 2: A systematic review of several studies examined the long-term effectiveness of the HCG diet. The results showed that the HCG diet resulted in significant weight loss, which was maintained after several months. In addition, positive changes were noted in waist circumference, blood pressure, and blood glucose levels. The study suggests that the HCG diet can achieve long-term weight loss results.

- Study 3: A study investigated the influence of the HCG diet on metabolism and body composition in women. The results showed that the HCG diet led to increased fat burning and boosted metabolism. In addition, improved insulin sensitivity was noted, indicating better regulation of blood glucose levels. The study suggests that the HCG diet may play a role not only in weight loss, but also in improving metabolism.

Overall, these studies show that the HCG diet is a promising approach to weight loss. The results suggest that the diet can be effective for losing weight, boosting metabolism, and improving body composition. However, it is important to note that individual results may vary and that the HCG diet is not suitable for everyone.

It is advisable to consult a qualified doctor or nutritionist before starting the HCG diet and to consider individual needs and health aspects. By working with an expert, you can ensure that the HCG diet best suits your goals and your body.

It remains to be emphasized that research on the HCG diet is still ongoing and new findings are being made. As a reader of this guide, it is important to keep up to date with current studies and research in order to make informed decisions and achieve the best possible results.

14.3 Comparison of the HCG diet with other dietary approaches

In this chapter, we will compare the HCG diet with other popular diet approaches to help you decide which approach is best for you. It is important to note that each person has individual needs and preferences, so there can be no "one size fits all" solution. Here are some important aspects to consider when comparing the HCG diet to other diet approaches:

- Weight loss: The HCG diet has proven to be effective for losing weight quickly. The focus is on a low-calorie diet and support from HCG hormones. Other diet approaches may also result in weight loss, but the speed and extent of weight loss may vary.
- Metabolism: An important advantage of the HCG diet is its influence on the metabolism. The combination of a specific diet and the use of HCG hormones boosts the metabolism, which can lead to increased fat burning and improved energy metabolism. Some other diet approaches may result in a slower metabolism.

- Sustainability: The HCG diet is primarily designed as a short-term diet to lose weight quickly. It is recommended to maintain a healthy diet and active lifestyle long-term after the diet to maintain weight loss. Other dietary approaches may be better integrated into a long-term sustainable lifestyle.
- Feeling hungry: A common concern with diets is the feeling of hunger. In the HCG diet, the combination of the specific diet and the HCG hormone intake reduces the feeling of hunger. In other diet approaches, the feeling of hunger may vary.
- Individuality: Everyone is unique, so certain diet approaches may suit a person better than others. It is important to consider your personal preferences, lifestyle and goals to find the most suitable approach for yourself.

Ultimately, it is up to you to evaluate your options and make an informed decision. It may also be helpful to speak with a qualified physician or dietitian for individualized advice and to address any concerns you may have. Remember that long-term weight loss and a healthy lifestyle require more than just dieting. It's about making lasting changes to your diet and lifestyle to achieve long-term results and improve your well-being.

14.4 Expert opinions and controversies about the HCG diet

In this chapter we would like to look at the expert opinions and controversial aspects of the HCG diet. It is important to understand that there are different opinions and viewpoints about this diet. Here are some expert opinions and controversies that are discussed in relation to the HCG diet:

- Expert Opinions: Some experts support the HCG diet and emphasize its effectiveness in rapid weight loss. They emphasize the benefits of a low-calorie diet and argue that HCG hormones can boost metabolism and promote fat loss.
- Scientific controversies: There are also experts and research results that question the effectiveness of the HCG diet. Some studies show that weight loss on the HCG diet is mainly due to the low-calorie diet and not the HCG hormones themselves. These

researchers argue that the HCG hormones have no significant effect on weight loss.

- Safety concerns: Another controversial issue is the potential risks and side effects of the HCG diet. Some experts warn that the diet is very low in calories, especially if done for a long period of time. It is recommended to follow the HCG diet under medical supervision to minimize potential risks.
- Long-term results: Another discussion concerns the long-term results of the HCG diet. Some experts emphasize that it is important to maintain a healthy lifestyle after the diet to maintain weight loss. They argue that long-term weight control cannot be achieved by the HCG diet alone.

It is important to note that the HCG diet is perceived differently by individuals and may not be suitable for everyone. It is recommended to talk to a qualified doctor or nutritionist before starting the diet to make an informed decision. You can also research various sources and information to get a comprehensive picture.

In conclusion, it is critical that you prioritize your own health and well-being. Take time to evaluate your options and choose the one that best suits you and your goals. It's also important to take a holistic approach to weight loss that includes healthy eating, regular physical activity and a balanced lifestyle.

14.5 Future developments and potential of the HCG diet

In this chapter, we take a look into the future and consider the potential developments of the HCG diet. Although the HCG diet has been around for some time, there is still room for further research and possible innovation. Here are some areas where the HCG diet could be further developed:

- Personalized approaches: One promising development lies in personalized tailoring of the HCG diet. Genetic testing and metabolic assessments could be used to tailor the diet to each person's individual needs and preferences. This could lead to improved efficacy and better outcomes.
- Combination with other therapies: There is potential to combine the HCG diet with other therapeutic approaches to further optimize

weight loss. For example, combining it with certain medications or complementary treatments could have a synergistic effect and lead to more effective weight loss.

- Further development of accompanying programs: In addition to the diet itself, companion programs and support systems could be further developed. This may include improved mobile apps, online communities, and coaching programs that provide comprehensive guidance and support to participants.
- Long-term studies: Future research could focus more on long-term studies to better understand the long-term success of the HCG diet. This could help to more accurately evaluate the long-term effects and ability of the HCG diet to maintain weight loss.
- Education and awareness: Another important development lies in the education and awareness of the HCG diet. By providing comprehensive and sound information, misunderstandings and misinformation can be avoided. This could help people make better informed decisions.

It is important to note that these potential developments are still under research and development and further studies are needed to confirm their efficacy and safety. It is advisable to stay abreast of the latest research and seek advice from qualified professionals to make informed decisions.

In conclusion, the HCG diet is a promising approach to weight loss that continues to be researched and developed. With the right information and a sound approach, you may be able to use the HCG diet effectively to achieve your weight loss goals.

Chapter 15: Conclusion and outlook

It has been demonstrated that the HCG diet is an all-encompassing method for achieving successful weight loss. In this book, we have discussed the fundamentals of the HCG diet, including its stages and benefits, as well as presented a wide range of suggestions, techniques, and recommendations for successfully implementing the diet. According to what we have seen, the HCG diet speeds up the metabolism, encourages fat reduction, and reduces the amount of muscle that is lost.

Not only is the HCG diet not a short-term solution, but it is also an all-encompassing method for achieving and maintaining weight management and sustained weight loss. Obtaining remarkable outcomes is possible with the utilization of HCG pills in conjunction with a diet low in calories and a healthy way of life. On the other hand, it is essential to keep in mind that the HCG diet is not appropriate for everyone, and that one must take into account their own requirements as well as any existing medical conditions.

The countless success stories of people who have participated in the HCG diet demonstrate that this strategy is effective and has the potential to bring about great results. There is a possibility that the HCG diet may not only help you lose weight, but it will also help you feel more confident in yourself and enhance your overall health.

On the other hand, it is essential to stress that the HCG diet is not a miracle cure and that it ought to be examined within the framework of a more full assessment. In order to maintain a healthy weight and maintain health over the long term, it is essential to have a balanced diet, engage in regular physical activity, get enough sleep, and learn how to manage stress.

In terms of the future of the HCG diet, there are developments and study results that are encouraging, which gives optimism for additional progress and changes to be made. Personalization of the diet, integration with other treatment modalities, and the utilization of contemporary technologies are only some of the areas that will be the subject of research and development in the years to come.

It is essential to acquire comprehensive information, consult with a medical professional, and arrive at a conclusion that is well-informed before to beginning the HCG diet. Individual requirements should always be taken into consideration because every body is different. It is possible to overcome potential obstacles and increase the likelihood of long-term success by receiving enough care and support while on the diet.

In conclusion, the HCG diet is an all-encompassing guide to efficient weight loss that has assisted a wide range of individuals in accomplishing their objectives concerning weight loss. The HCG diet has the potential to be an effective method for encouraging a healthy lifestyle and getting rid of excess weight if it is approached with the appropriate mindset, the appropriate information, and a customized approach.